Spinal Infections

Editor

E. TURGUT TALI

NEUROIMAGING CLINICS
OF NORTH AMERICA

www.neuroimaging.theclinics.com

Consulting Editor
SURESH K. MUKHERJI

May 2015 • Volume 25 • Number 2

ELSEVIER

1600 John F. Kennedy Boulevard • Suite 1800 • Philadelphia, Pennsylvania, 19103-2899

http://www.neuroimaging.theclinics.com

NEUROIMAGING CLINICS OF NORTH AMERICA Volume 25, Number 2
May 2015 ISSN 1052-5149, ISBN 13: 978-0-323-37609-9

Editor: John Vassallo (j.vassallo@elsevier.com)
Developmental Editor: Casey Jackson

Neuroimaging Clinics of North America (ISSN 1052-5149) is published quarterly by Elsevier Inc., 360 Park Avenue South, New York, NY 10010-1710. Months of issue are February, May, August, and November. Business and editorial offices: 1600 John F. Kennedy Blvd., Suite 1800, Philadelphia, PA 19103-2899. Business and editorial offices: 6277 Sea Harbor Drive, Orlando, FL 32887-4800. Periodicals postage paid at New York, NY, and additional mailing offices. Subscription prices are USD 360 per year for US individuals, USD 514 per year for US institutions, USD 180 per year for US students and residents, USD 415 per year for Canadian individuals, USD 655 per year for Canadian institutions, USD 525 per year for international individuals, USD 655 per year for international institutions and USD 260 per year for Canadian and foreign students and residents. To receive student/resident rate, orders must be accompanied by name of affiliated institution, date of term, and the *signature* of program/residency coordinator on institution letterhead. Orders will be billed at individual rate until proof of status is received. Foreign air speed delivery is included in all *Clinics* subscription prices. All prices are subject to change without notice. POSTMASTER: Send address changes to *Neuroimaging Clinics of North America*, Elsevier Health Sciences Division, Subscription Customer Service, 3251 Riverport Lane, Maryland Heights, MO 63043. Telephone: 1-800-654-2452 (U.S. and Canada); 314-447-8871 (outside U.S. and Canada). Fax: 314-447-8029. E-mail: journalscustomerservice-usa@elsevier.com (for print support); journalsonlinesupport-usa@elsevier.com (for online support).

Reprints. For copies of 100 or more of articles in this publication, please contact the Commercial Reprints Department, Elsevier Inc., 360 Park Avenue South, New York, NY 10010-1710. Tel.: 212-633-3874; Fax: 212-633-3820; E-mail: reprints@elsevier.com.

Neuroimaging Clinics of North America is covered by *Excerpta Medical/EMBASE,* the RSNA Index of Imaging Literature, *MEDLINE/PubMed (Index Medicus),* MEDLINE/MEDLARS, SciSearch, Research Alert, and Neuroscience Citation Index.

PROGRAM OBJECTIVE

The goal of *Neuroimaging Clinics of North America* is to keep practicing radiologists and radiology residents up to date with current clinical practice in radiology by providing timely articles reviewing the state of the art in patient care.

TARGET AUDIENCE

Practicing radiologists, radiology residents, and other healthcare professionals who utilize neuroimaging findings to provide patient care.

LEARNING OBJECTIVES

Upon completion of this activity, participants will be able to:
1. Review imaging and other diagnostic techniques in pediatric spinal infections.
2. Discuss the pathological basis of pediatric spinal infections.
3. Recognize treatments and complications in pediatric spinal infections.

ACCREDITATION

The Elsevier Office of Continuing Medical Education (EOCME) is accredited by the Accreditation Council for Continuing Medical Education (ACCME) to provide continuing medical education for physicians.

The EOCME designates this enduring material for a maximum of 15 *AMA PRA Category 1 Credit*(s)™. Physicians should claim only the credit commensurate with the extent of their participation in the activity.

All other health care professionals requesting continuing education credit for this enduring material will be issued a certificate of participation.

DISCLOSURE OF CONFLICTS OF INTEREST

The EOCME assesses conflict of interest with its instructors, faculty, planners, and other individuals who are in a position to control the content of CME activities. All relevant conflicts of interest that are identified are thoroughly vetted by EOCME for fair balance, scientific objectivity, and patient care recommendations. EOCME is committed to providing its learners with CME activities that promote improvements or quality in healthcare and not a specific proprietary business or a commercial interest.

The planning committee, staff, authors and editors listed below have identified no financial relationships or relationships to products or devices they or their spouse/life partner have with commercial interest related to the content of this CME activity:

Selim Ayhan, MD; Frank De Belder, MD; Sally Candy, MBChB, FcRad (Diag) SA; Antonio Jose da Rocha, MD, PhD; Federico D'Orazio, MD; Guldal Esendagli-Yilmaz, MD; Lázaro Luís Faria do Amaral, MD; Marguerite Faure, MD; Anjali Fortna; Massimo Gallucci, MD; Kristen Helm; Derya Burcu Hazer, MD; Renato Hoffmann Nunes, MD; Jef Huyskens, MD; Tracy Kilborn, MBChB, FRCR (UK); A. Murat Koc, MD; Suresh K. Mukherji, MD, MBA, FACR; A. Yusuf Oner, MD; Selcuk Palaoglu, MD; Paul M. Parizel, MD, PhD; Andrea Rossi, MD; Karthikeyan Subramaniam; E. Turgut Tali, MD; Tarik Tihan, MD, PhD; Omer Uluoglu, MD; Luc van den Hauwe, MD; Johan Van Goethem, MD, PhD; Pieter Janse van Rensburg, MBChB, FRCR (UK), MMed (RadDiag), FRCPC; John Vassallo; Caroline Venstermans, MD; Hajime Yokota, MD, PhD.

The planning committee, staff, authors and editors listed below have identified financial relationships or relationships to products or devices they or their spouse/life partner have with commercial interest related to the content of this CME activity:

Kei Yamada, MD, PhD is a consultant/advisor at Lundbeck, and has research support from Daichi Sankyo Company, Limited; Bayer AG; Eisai Co., Ltd.; Nihon Medi-Physics Co., Ltd.; Siemens AG; and The Termo Company.

UNAPPROVED/OFF-LABEL USE DISCLOSURE

The EOCME requires CME faculty to disclose to the participants:
1. When products or procedures being discussed are off-label, unlabelled, experimental, and/or investigational (not US Food and Drug Administration [FDA] approved); and
2. Any limitations on the information presented, such as data that are preliminary or that represent ongoing research, interim analyses, and/or unsupported opinions. Faculty may discuss information about pharmaceutical agents that is outside of FDA-approved labelling. This information is intended solely for CME and is not intended to promote off-label use of these medications. If you have any questions, contact the medical affairs department of the manufacturer for the most recent prescribing information.

TO ENROLL

To enroll in the *Neuroimaging Clinics of North America* Continuing Medical Education program, call customer service at 1-800-654-2452 or sign up online at http://www.theclinics.com/home/cme. The CME program is available to subscribers for an additional annual fee of USD 235.

METHOD OF PARTICIPATION

In order to claim credit, participants must complete the following:

1. Complete enrolment as indicated above.
2. Read the activity.
3. Complete the CME Test and Evaluation. Participants must achieve a score of 70% on the test. All CME Tests and Evaluations must be completed online.

CME INQUIRIES/SPECIAL NEEDS

For all CME inquiries or special needs, please contact elsevierCME@elsevier.com.

NEUROIMAGING CLINICS OF NORTH AMERICA

THE CLINICS ARE AVAILABLE ONLINE!
Access your subscription at:
www.theclinics.com

Contributors

CONSULTING EDITOR

SURESH K. MUKHERJI, MD, MBA, FACR
Professor and Chairman; Walter F. Patenge
Endowed Chair, Department of Radiology;
Chief Medical Officer and Director, Michigan
State University Health Team, Michigan State
University, East Lansing, Michigan

EDITOR

E. TURGUT TALI, MD
Professor and Chair, Division of
Neuroradiology, Department of Radiology,
Gazi University School of Medicine, Ankara,
Turkey

AUTHORS

SELIM AYHAN, MD
Specialist in Neurosurgery, Department of
Neurosurgery, Malatya State Hospital,
Malatya, Turkey

SALLY CANDY, MBChB, FcRad (Diag) SA
Department of Radiology, Groote Schuur
Hospital, University of Cape Town, Cape Town,
South Africa

FEDERICO D'ORAZIO, MD
Neuroradiology Unit, S. Salvatore Hospital,
L'Aquila, Italy

ANTONIO JOSE DA ROCHA, MD, PhD
Division of Neuroradiology, Santa Casa de
Misericórdia de São Paulo; Division of
Neuroradiology, Fleury Medicina e Saúde,
São Paulo, São Paulo, Brazil

FRANK DE BELDER, MD
Department of Radiology, Antwerp University
Hospital, University of Antwerp, Edegem,
Belgium

GULDAL ESENDAGLI-YILMAZ, MD
Associate Professor, Department of Medical
Pathology, Faculty of Medicine, Gazi
University, Ankara, Turkey

LÁZARO LUÍS FARIA DO AMARAL, MD
Division of Neuroradiology, Santa Casa de
Misericórdia de São Paulo; Division of
Neuroradiology, MEDIMAGEM - Hospital da
Beneficência Portuguesa de São Paulo, São
Paulo, São Paulo, Brazil

MARGUERITE FAURE, MD
Department of Radiology, Antwerp University
Hospital, University of Antwerp, Edegem,
Belgium

Prof MASSIMO GALLUCCI, MD
President of the Italian Association of
Neuroradiology, Diagnostic and Interventional
(AINR); Professor and Chairman of
Neuroradiology, Head of Neuroradiology Unit,
S. Salvatore Hospital, University of L'Aquila,
L'Aquila, Italy

DERYA BURCU HAZER, MD
Associate Professor, Department of
Neurosurgery, Mugla Sitki Kocman University
School of Medicine, Mugla, Turkey

JEF HUYSKENS, MD
Department of Radiology, Antwerp University
Hospital, University of Antwerp, Edegem,
Belgium

TRACY KILBORN, MBChB, FRCR (UK)
Department of Pediatric Radiology, Red Cross
War Memorial Children's Hospital, University of
Cape Town, Cape Town, South Africa

A. MURAT KOC, MD
Fellow, Department of Radiology, Gazi
University School of Medicine, Ankara, Turkey

RENATO HOFFMANN NUNES, MD
Division of Neuroradiology, Santa Casa de
Misericórdia de São Paulo; Division of
Neuroradiology, Fleury Medicina e Saúde,
São Paulo, São Paulo, Brazil

A. YUSUF ONER, MD
Professor of Radiology, Neuroradiology
Division, Department of Radiology, Gazi
University School of Medicine, Ankara, Turkey

SELCUK PALAOGLU, MD, PhD
Professor of Neurosurgery, Department of
Neurosurgery, Hacettepe University School of
Medicine, Ankara, Turkey

PAUL M. PARIZEL, MD, PhD
Department of Radiology, Antwerp University
Hospital, University of Antwerp, Edegem,
Belgium

ANDREA ROSSI, MD
Department of Pediatric Neuroradiology,
Istituto Giannina Gaslini, Genova, Italy

E. TURGUT TALI, MD
Professor and Chair, Division of
Neuroradiology, Department of Radiology,
Gazi University School of Medicine, Ankara,
Turkey

TARIK TIHAN, MD, PhD
Professor, Neuropathology Division,
Department of Pathology, University of
California San Francisco, San Francisco,
California; Visiting Professor, Koc
University School of Medicine, Istanbul,
Turkey

OMER ULUOGLU, MD
Professor, Department of Medical Pathology,
Faculty of Medicine, Gazi University, Ankara,
Turkey

LUC VAN DEN HAUWE, MD
Department of Radiology, Antwerp University
Hospital, University of Antwerp, Edegem,
Belgium

JOHAN VAN GOETHEM, MD, PhD
Department of Radiology, Antwerp University
Hospital, University of Antwerp, Edegem,
Belgium

**PIETER JANSE VAN RENSBURG, MBChB,
FRCR (UK), MMed (RadDiag), FRCPC**
Department of Medical Imaging, Regina
General Hospital, College of Medicine,
University of Saskatchewan, Regina,
Canada

CAROLINE VENSTERMANS, MD
Department of Radiology, Antwerp University
Hospital, University of Antwerp, Edegem,
Belgium

KEI YAMADA, MD, PhD
Department of Radiology, Graduate School of
Medical Science, Kyoto Prefectural University
of Medicine, Kyoto, Japan

HAJIME YOKOTA, MD, PhD
Department of Radiology, Graduate
School of Medical Science, Kyoto
Prefectural University of Medicine, Kyoto,
Japan; Department of Diagnostic Radiology
and Radiation Oncology, Graduate
School of Medicine, Chiba University,
Chiba, Japan

Contents

> Pyogenic spondylitis and discitis are usually seen following a recent infection or surgery. A septic embolus causes an infarcted area within the bone. Pyogenic spondylitis is characterized by edema, vascular leakage, and supportive inflammatory reaction characterized with polymorphonuclear leukocytes. In tuberculosis of the spine, active lesions are characterized by formation of epithelioid granulomas with central caseating necrosis. *Mycobacterium tuberculosis* can be shown by histochemical stains for acid-fast bacteria or by immunochemistry. In brucella spondylitis, microgranulomatous proliferation composed of histiocytes containing numerous bacilli without caseating necrosis is characteristic. *Brucella melitensis* can be shown on histochemical Gram stain.

> The pathologic evaluation of spinal cord infections requires comprehensive clinical, radiological, and laboratory correlation, because the histologic findings in acute, chronic, or granulomatous infections rarely provide clues for the specific cause. This brief review focuses on the pathologic mechanisms as well as practical issues in the diagnosis and reporting of infections of the spinal cord. Examples are provided of the common infectious agents and methods for their diagnosis. By necessity, discussion is restricted to the infections of the medulla spinalis proper and its meninges, and not bone or soft tissue infections.

> Inflammatory and infectious disorders of the spine in children are less common than in adults, and are usually categorized according to location into (1) those predominantly affecting the spinal cord; (2) those predominantly affecting the nerve roots and meninges; and (3) those predominantly affecting the vertebrae, discs, and epidural space. Magnetic resonance imaging with contrast material administration is of paramount importance for an adequate identification and characterization of these disorders.

> Spinal infections are a spectrum of disease comprising spondylitis, diskitis, spondylodiskitis, pyogenic facet arthropathy, epidural infections, meningitis, polyradiculopathy, and myelitis. Inflammation can be caused by pyogenic, granulomatous, autoimmune,

idiopathic, and iatrogenic conditions. In an era of immune suppression, tuberculosis, and HIV epidemic, together with worldwide socioeconomic fluctuations, spinal infections are increasing. Despite advanced diagnostic technology, diagnosis of this entity and differentiation from degenerative disease, noninfective inflammatory lesions, and spinal neoplasms are difficult. Radiological evaluations play an important role, along with contrast-enhanced MR imaging the modality of choice in diagnosis, evaluation, treatment planning, interventional treatment, and treatment monitoring of spinal infections.

The prevalence of tuberculosis (TB) has increased in developing and developed countries as a consequence of the AIDS epidemic, immigration, social deprivation, and inadequate TB control and screening programs. Spinal TB may be osseous or nonosseous. Classic findings of multiple contiguous vertebral body involvement, gibbus formation, and subligamentous spread with paravertebral abscesses are optimally evaluated with MR imaging. Nonspondylitic spinal TB is less well-described in the literature, may develop in the absence of TB meningitis, and is often associated with meningovascular cord ischemia. Radiologists should be familiar with the spectrum of imaging findings, allowing early diagnosis and treatment of this serious condition.

Spinal involvement in human brucellosis is a common condition and a significant cause of morbidity and mortality, particularly in endemic areas, because it is often associated with therapeutic failure. Most chronic brucellosis cases are the result of inadequate treatment of the initial episode. Recognition of spinal brucellosis is challenging. Early diagnosis is important to ensure proper treatment and decrease morbidity and mortality. Radiologic evaluation has gained importance in diagnosis and treatment planning, including interventional procedures and monitoring of all spinal infections.

This article summarizes myelopathy and radiculopathy caused by different viruses. The cases described are divided into three categories: acute myelitis and radiculitis, postinfectious myelopathy and radiculopathy, and chronic myelopathy. Some diseases present with characteristic imaging findings. For example, varicella zoster virus tends to injure the dorsal column, whereas poliovirus tends to injure the frontal horns. Magnetic resonance imaging is an essential tool in diagnosis. However, because imaging findings are often nonspecific, consideration of a combination of diagnostic procedures, including the clinical course, symptoms, and laboratory data, is necessary for making a correct diagnosis.

The imaging features of spinal parasitic diseases and other rare infections are herein discussed. These diseases are distributed worldwide, with increased prevalence in areas with poor sanitary conditions and in developing countries. In nonendemic areas, sporadic cases may occur, consequent to increased international travel and immunocompromising conditions. Infectious diseases are usually treatable, and early detection is often crucial. A thorough comprehension of the imaging patterns associated with the clinical features, epidemiology, and laboratory results allows the radiologist to narrow down the options for differential diagnosis and facilitates the timely implementation of appropriate therapies.

Spinal infections are challenging to diagnose and represent a life-threatening medical condition. Diagnosis is often delayed because of nonspecific accompanying symptoms. The role of interventional neuroradiology in spinal infection is double: diagnostic and therapeutic, consisting substantially of 2 main procedures, represented by spine biopsies and positioning of percutaneous drainage, which represent a minimally invasive, faster and more cost-effective alternative to open surgery procedures. This article will focus on the available state-of-the-art techniques to perform discovertebral image-guided biopsies in case of suspected infections and on image-guided placement of percutaneous drainage to treat infectious collections of the spine and paravertebral structures.

Spinal infection is rare. Clinical suspicion is important in patients with nonmechanical neck and/or back pain to make the proper diagnosis in early disease. Before planning surgery, a thorough evaluation of the spinal stability, alignment, and deformity is necessary. Timing of surgery, side of approach, appropriate surgical technique, and spinal instruments used are crucial. Biomechanical preservation of the spinal column during and after the infection is a significant issue. Postoperative spine infection is another entity of which spinal surgeons should be aware of. Proper septic conditions with meticulous planning of surgery are essential for successful spine surgery and better outcome.

Spondylitis or infection of the spine is a spectrum of diseases involving the bone, disks, and/or ligaments. Because of a significant increase in the immunocompromised patient population, spinal infections are a growing and changing group of conditions, making the diagnosis based on imaging more challenging. Most cases of spinal infections are pyogenic and occur after hematogeneous spread of an infection located elsewhere in the body. A prompt diagnosis remains crucial and MR imaging remains the cornerstone in the diagnosis. This article provides a pictorial overview of the complications and sequelae in spinal infections in general. Discussed are postoperative infections, extraspinal spread of infection, fractures and malformations, and neurologic complications.

Foreword
Spinal Infections

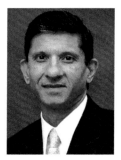

Suresh K. Mukherji, MD, MBA, FACR
Consulting Editor

This issue of the *Neuroimaging Clinics* focuses on the complex subject of spinal infections. It is important for radiologists to be aware of various imaging features of spinal infections and distinguish them from degenerative inflammatory, metabolic, and neoplastic diseases. This issue reviews the role of imaging in spinal infections and provides the latest information on the pathophysiologic basis of various spinal infections. There are dedicated articles on interventional procedures, surgical treatments, and complications. There is also an article specifically devoted to pediatric spinal infections.

The guest editor of this issue deserves special notice. Turgo Tali is a world-renowned neuroradiologist, who was President of the highly successful XXth Symposium Neuroradiologicum. I am very honored to call him a friend and thank him and all of the article authors for taking time from their very busy schedules to produce such an outstanding issue.

Suresh K. Mukherji, MD, MBA, FACR
Michigan State University Health Team
Department of Radiology
Michigan State University
846 Service Road
East Lansing, MI 48824, USA

E-mail address:
mukherji@rad.msu.edu

http://dx.doi.org/10.1016/j.nic.2015.02.002
1052-5149/15/$ – see front matter © 2015 Published by Elsevier Inc.

neuroimaging.theclinics.com

Preface
Spinal Infection

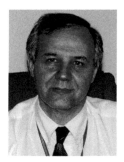

E. Turgut Tali, MD
Editor

This issue of the *Neuroimaging Clinics* focuses on spinal infections as one of the most significant causes of morbidity and even mortality involving the nervous system. Differentiation of spinal infections from degenerative processes, inflammatory disorders, metabolic disorders, and neoplasms is still challenging even with the dazzling development of diagnostic tools. Early and accurate diagnosis of spinal infections and differentiation from these disorders, which have different treatments, are essential to decrease morbidity, mainly neurologic complications that reduce the quality of life, increasing health care costs. Radiologic evaluations together with interventional procedures have gained importance in the diagnosis, treatment planning, treatment, and monitoring of spinal infections. Interventional procedures ranging from biopsy to minimally invasive treatments are also introduced for the benefit of the physicians who care for patients with spinal infections in both private practice and academia.

Spinal infections may show different imaging features according to the host's immune status, current or prior medication (particularly antimicrobial agents and steroids), infecting agent, endemic and geographic differences, and so on. It is important for radiologists to become aware of these different features, mainly atypical signal intensity alterations and contrast enhancement patterns on magnetic resonance imaging of spinal infections, so as not to exclude infection when some of the typical signs are lacking for the diagnosis.

The outstanding contributions in this issue describe the current role of imaging in spinal infections, detailing what is currently known regarding the pathophysiologic and histopathologic basis, minimally invasive-interventional procedures, surgical treatments, complications, and sequelae formation. We tried to present to the readers detailed information that they can apply in providing a thoughtful assessment and perspective in their practice.

As guest editor, I have been fortunate to have colleagues willing to share their knowledge and expertise for this issue. I personally express my sincere gratitude to all the authors for their excellent contributions.

We hope this issue will be helpful, informative, and educational in understanding spinal infections.

E. Turgut Tali, MD
Professor and Chair
Division of Neuroradiology
Department of Radiology
Gazi University School of Medicine
Besevler, Ankara 06560
Turkey

E-mail address:
turgut.tali@gmail.com

http://dx.doi.org/10.1016/j.nic.2015.02.001
1052-5149/15/$ – see front matter © 2015 Published by Elsevier Inc.

neuroimaging.theclinics.com

Pathologic Basis of Pyogenic, Nonpyogenic, and Other Spondylitis and Discitis

Guldal Esendagli-Yilmaz, MD*, Omer Uluoglu, MD

KEYWORDS

- Spondylitis • Discitis • Spondylodiscitis • Tuberculosis

KEY POINTS

- Histopathologic features should be correlated with the pathologic changes during the evaluation of different stages of spondylitis with various causes.
- Differential diagnosis between pyogenic and chronic granulomatous spondylitis is significant for the outcome of the patients.
- Histopathologic changes seen in discitis, although primarily less investigated, could be helpful for understanding the nature of the disease.

PYOGENIC SPONDYLITIS AND DISCITIS

Pyogenic spondylitis and discitis are usually seen following a recent infection or a surgery. In routine practice, because vertebral osteomyelitis and intervertebral discitis usually occur in conjunction with one another, spondylodiscitis is the preferred term to define this condition. The most common cause of both pyogenic spondylitis and discitis is hematogenous spread of Staphylococcus aureus.

In adults, the intervertebral disc is avascular, without direct blood supply; in contrast, the subchondral metaphyseal region of the vertebral body has the richest vascular network. A septic embolus causes an infarcted area within the bone where a subsequent infection settles down to form pyogenic spondylitis. As well as many other enzymes, the pyogenic bacteria express some receptors for collagen, the main bone matrix component, which help them to adhere.[1]

Most hematogenous infections of the disc space are the result of dissemination from the infected adjacent bone. However, in isolated discitis, inoculation of the pyogenic bacteria during the surgical procedure under suboptimal conditions remains the main cause. Here, the protease activity via proteolytic enzymes of pyogenic bacteria is particularly responsible for degrading of proteins within the disc structure.[1]

Pyogenic spondylitis is characterized by a suppurative inflammatory reaction. Within the infected area, histologic changes are closely related to the duration of spondylitis. In the early acute phase, vascular dilation and vascular endothelial fluid leakage produce edema between the intertrabecular area of bone. The vessels in the bone marrow are fenestrated, enabling the rapid fluid outflow. The pressure of the area increases and the vascular blood flow reduces, initiating the ischemic process. The acute inflammatory exudate composed of polymorphonuclear cells, mainly the neutrophil leukocytes, and proteinous material then collects in this infected area. Because the bone is highly vascularized,

Disclosures: None.
Department of Medical Pathology, Faculty of Medicine, Gazi University, Yenimahalle, Ankara 06500, Turkey
* Corresponding author.
E-mail address: drguldal@yahoo.com

ischemia-induced endogenous lysosomal activity of neutrophils destroys the bone matrix more rapidly. Because of this suppuration and ongoing ischemia, bone necrosis develops within 48 hours. If the inflamed area is close to the cortex, cortical bone destruction may be prominent, otherwise the destruction mainly takes place in the medulla.

In discitis, especially when the disc has a degenerative disease or a traumatic condition, which means a vascularized disc structure facilitating these enzymatic activities, the progression of this acute inflammatory phase is more rapid. In the subacute and early regenerative phases, after the first 48 hours, the neutrophilic infiltration gradually ceases and mononuclear inflammatory cells (mainly the lymphocytes and macrophages) enter the area within the granulation tissue made up of newly formed fine capillary network and proliferation of fibroblastic cells in an edematous background. This process results in swelling of the disc. The degenerative and destructive changes characterized by a cracking and myxohyalinized appearance follow this stage. In the late regenerative and subsequent chronic phase, edema subsides, lymphocytes and plasma cells dominate, and fibroblastic proliferation accompanies, which may end up the shrinked and sclerotic disc material.

The elastase activity of *Staphylococcus aureus* destroys the elastic reticular network of the bone and the discs, particularly inducing fibrosis. However, even in the chronic stage, neutrophil foci may continue to exist, as well as areas of ischemic necrosis and reactive newly produced bone.[1]

SUBACUTE AND CHRONIC SPONDYLITIS

Subacute and chronic spondylitis are frequently associated with tuberculosis[2,3] and, to a lesser extent, brucellosis[2,4] and fungal infections.[5] In tuberculosis of the spine (Pott disease), active lesions are characterized by formation of granulomas mainly made up of epithelioid histiocytes with central caseating necrosis. These granulomas tend to come together to form a larger conglomerated appearance. These granulomas are surrounded by a fibroblastic ring containing many lymphocytes. Typical Langhans-type multinuclear giant cells are scattered within granulomas or are peripherally located. In immunocompromised patients, the fibroblastic ring is not well developed and lymphocyte infiltration is poor.

In late phases, granulomas may be replaced by fibrous tissue and dystrophic calcifications may be seen. *Mycobacterium tuberculosis* can be shown by histochemical stains for acid-fast bacteria or by immunochemistry in early exudative and caseating phases, whereas in the late fibrocalcifying stages it is almost impossible to do so. In addition, beginning in the early phases, spreading of the inflammation and bone necrosis develops, giving rise to ischemia, pathologic fractures, and sequestrate formation.

In brucella spondylitis, microgranulomatous proliferation composed of histiocytes containing numerous bacilli without caseating necrosis is characteristic. Those gram-negative bacilli can be shown on histochemical Gram stain.[6] In contrast with pyogenic bacteria, the major pathogen in human brucellosis, *Brucella melitensis*, does not contain proteinase activity to destroy the collagenous matrix, which partly explains why the intervertebral disc, although not primarily involved, is entrapped within exudative material and why diffuse reactive bone marrow changes characterized by myxoedematous changes is seen without bone destruction. As a basic mechanism in bone turnover, osteoclasts are principally affected by osteoblasts via growth factors, so there is a continuum of lysis, proliferation, and sclerosis during the infectious process. Osteoclasts are specialized macrophages; they are destroyers of the bone matrix, and are mainly located in spongious areas and in the endosteal surface of the bone. When they are activated by infectious stimuli, they transform into epithelioid histiocytes and use nitric oxide via the NADPH (nicotinamide adenine dinucleotide phosphate hydrogen) pathway to kill the microorganism. In brucella spondylitis, osteoblastic activity is induced and this may partly explain the diffuse inflammation pattern of brucella spondylodiscitis without prominent bone and disc destruction. Because both *Mycobacterium* and *Brucella* are intracellular bacilli, they induce less exudative reaction and the main limiting agent is the macrophage response associated by the immunocompetence of the patient. Also, following subacute or chronic granulomatous spondylodiscitis, histopathologic features of tissue regeneration do not correlate with the clinical or the radiological findings during the healing phase. In fungal spondylodiscitis, which is rare and mainly affects immunocompromised patients, the fungal hyphae showing the differential branching features are usually seen within the lesion, on histology with routine hematoxylin and eosin or histochemical silver stains.

REFERENCES

1. Rosenberg AE. Bones, joints, and soft-tissue tumors. In: Kumar V, Abbas AK, Fausto N, et al, editors. Robbins and Cotran pathologic basis of disease. 8th edition. Philadelphia: Saunders Elsevier; 2010. p. 1221–3.

2. Turunc T, Demiroglu YZ, Uncu H, et al. A comparative analysis of tuberculous, brucellar and pyogenic spontaneous spondylodiscitis patients. J Infect 2007;55(2):158–63.

3. Pertuiset E, Beaudreuil J, Liote F, et al. Spinal tuberculosis in adults. A study of 103 cases in a developed country, 1998–1994. Medicine (Baltimore) 1999;78(5):309–20.

4. Colmenero JD, Reguera JM, Martos F, et al. Complications associated with Brucella melitensis infection: a study of 530 cases. Medicine (Baltimore) 1996;75(4):195–211. Available at: http://www.ncbi.nlm.nih.gov/pubmed/?term=Causse%20M%5BAuthor%5D&cauthor=true&cauthor_uid=8699960.

5. Kim CW, Perry A, Currier B, et al. Fungal infections of the spine. Clin Orthop Relat Res 2006;444:92–9.

6. Araj GF. Human brucellosis: a classical infectious disease with persistent diagnostic challenges. Clin Lab Sci 1999;12(4):207–12.

Pathologic Approach to Spinal Cord Infections

Tarik Tihan, MD, PhD[a,b,*]

KEYWORDS

- Abscess • Bacteria • Fungus • Granuloma • Infections • Meningitis • Myelitis • Myelopathy

KEY POINTS

- Early suspicion of infectious cause with tissue biopsy at the appropriate stage is critical for correct identification and effective treatment of patients with infectious myelitis.
- Infections that diffusely involve the spinal meninges often coexist with involvement of the cranial meninges.
- Some infectious myelitides may not present with typical signs and symptoms of an infectious disease.
- The clinical practitioner should be aware of the infectious agents that can readily be recognized on a biopsy versus those that require stringent culturing and/or serologic analyses.
- Obtaining sufficient tissue for histologic recognition of the infectious agent in the spinal cord can be challenging, and planning should involve the pathologist.
- The use of biopsy or cytology material for detection of infectious agents should always be complemented by appropriately chosen microbiological cultures and serologic analyses.
- For infectious myelitides of unclear cause, more specialized analyses such as molecular testing may be useful in the diagnosis.

INTRODUCTION

Pathologic analysis of tissue can be performed to recognize the nature of the disease, help decide on the patient's management, or determine the efficacy of treatment.[1] These goals are also applicable for the infections of the spinal cord, myelitis, and myelomeningitis. This article focuses on the infectious agents that affect the parenchyma and the meninges of the spinal cord and their recognition.

Many infectious myelitides are iatrogenic or secondary, and many are associated with systemic infections. Predisposing factors include immunosuppression, immune deficiency syndromes as well as systemic inflammatory conditions such as lupus or collagen vascular diseases. Meningitis often coexists in the spinal and cranial meninges, which implies that the patients may present with focal neurologic deficits, cranial nerve dysfunction, constitutional symptoms and signs of infection, and/or symptoms and signs related to local destructive effects. In systemic infections, the neurologic findings are often preceded by a prodromal disease characterized by fever, headache, arthralgia, malaise, or confusion. Local abscess formation is also a more common presentation of some pathogens, such as tuberculosis. A sensory level can help localize the infectious process in the spinal cord, and acute presentations may involve urinary or bowel incontinence. Clinical and radiological information is critical to the pathologist for the appropriate workup of tissues from patients with spinal cord infections. A detailed clinical as well as

Disclosure: None.
[a] Neuropathology Division, Department of Pathology, University of California San Francisco, Room M551, 505 Parnassus Avenue, San Francisco, CA 94143-0102, USA; [b] Koc University School of Medicine, Istanbul, Turkey
* Neuropathology Division, Department of Pathology, University of California San Francisco, Room M551, 505 Parnassus Avenue, San Francisco, CA 94143-0102.
E-mail address: tarik.tihan@ucsf.edu

radiological assessment is beyond the scope of this article, but can be found in more comprehensive reviews on this matter.[2,3]

Principal pathologic analysis of infectious diseases includes a series of routine stains. The initial stage is a hematoxylin and eosin (H&E) stain, in which some infectious agents can be readily identified. Bacteria appear as uniform, hematoxyphilic clusters of rods or spheres much smaller than any cell. Fungal yeast and hyphae can also be identified, but some require special stains for identification. Inclusions of viral pathogens, such as cytomegalovirus (CMV), herpes simplex virus (HSV), and progressive multifocal leukoencephalopathy, are also recognized on H&E stains. Special stains include the Gram stain or its modifications, which are often the first step in identifying bacteria. These stains rely on the retention of crystal violet in the thick peptidoglycan cell wall of some bacteria and display a purple color, while the bacteria without this thick cell wall stain red with the safranin counterstain. Gomori or Grocott methenamine silver or modifications of this silver staining technique are often used to identify fungal organisms. Warthin-Starry staining method is used to detect spirochetes, whereas Ziehl-Nielsen and other similar methods are used in the identification of acid-fast bacilli such as tuberculosis. Other stains including periodic acid-Schiff (PAS) can also be used for identification of microorganisms, but the appropriate use of these special stains require sufficient clinical information and preliminary analysis of the H&E slides and should always be guided by the common sense of the pathologist.

CAUSES OF SPINAL CORD INFECTIONS
Bacterial Infections

Bacterial meningitis involving the spinal meninges are more common than spinal parenchymal infections and may be due to hematogenic spread of microorganisms or direct spread from an infectious source or may occur following surgery, trauma, and other manipulations.[4,5] On the other hand, myelitis is a rare manifestation or occurrence of bacterial infections. Most bacterial myelitis also involves the paraspinal soft tissues and/or the vertebrae. Most common bacterial pathogens for myelitis and spinal meningitis and their pathologic features are described below.

Streptococcus pneumoniae, Neisseria meningitidis, Haemophilus influenza, and *Listeria monocytogenes* are among the most common causes of meningitis in children as well as adults.[6] In the neonatal period, group B *Streptococci, Escherichia coli,*[7] and, in adults, gram-negative bacilli can be added to this list. These organisms more commonly involve the cranial meninges. In addition, many other species can be isolated from spinal meninges.[8–12] Common and uncommon pathogens are also reported as the cause of abscess and meningitis following surgery or trauma to the spinal cord.[5,10,11] Bacterial meningitis, especially streptococcal meningitides, can also be seen in the setting of immune deficiency, such as human immunodeficiency virus (HIV)/AIDS. Diabetes mellitus, surgical procedures, malignancies such as multiple myeloma, and liver disease are among the conditions that constitute risk factors for the development of meningitis. Inflammatory conditions, such as collagen vascular diseases or inflammatory bowel diseases, can also predispose to myelomeningitis and/or spinal cord abscesses.[13,14]

Histologically, the acute meningitides are characterized by an intense infiltration of polymorphonuclear leukocytes admixed with necrotic debris constituting the purulent material. Rarely, lymphocytes, macrophages, and plasma cells may also be observed. Special stains are most helpful in the acute inflammatory phase for the identification of intracellular or extracellular bacteria. Gram stain and its modifications are most useful in this phase when the neutrophilic infiltration is prominent.

Chronic meningitis can be caused by several bacterial pathogens that include *Mycobacteria* spp, *Treponema pallidum, Borrelia burgdorferii, Brucella abortus, L monocytogenes, Rickettsia* spp, *Chlamydia,* and *Bartonella henselae.*[15]

Detection and identification of bacteria in tissues can often be performed using routine Gram stains followed by microbiological tests or cultures. In some circumstances, tissue recognition even with special stains may not be possible and serologic testing, wherever available, can be useful in diagnosis. Serologic or DNA testing for brucella,[16] listeria,[17,18] rickettsia,[19] and other bacterial species can be used if there is sufficiently high suspicion clinically.

Tuberculosis incidence appears to be on the increase in some developed and developing countries, and there is an expanding number of mycobacterial species showing resistance to standard antibiotic treatment.[20] Tuberculous meningitis or myelitis is often a secondary extension from pulmonary or other primary sites.[21] One of the most common forms of myelopathy associated with tuberculosis is the tuberculous spondylitis, otherwise known as the Pott disease. The infection results in an abscess formation, compressing the spinal cord, and occasionally causing obstruction of the anterior spinal artery.[22,23] Occasionally, granulomatous inflammation associated with tuberculosis involves spinal meninges and parenchyma without bony involvement. Histologically, the destruction is due to well-formed granulomata with necrosis (ie, caseating granuloma) and multinucleated giant cells. The infectious process can involve any tissue type, including spinal cord parenchyma, meninges, disc and cartilage, soft tissue, and bone. Tissue diagnosis of tuberculosis can be made with the acid-fast stains such as Ziehl-Nielsen, Fite, Ellis-Zabrowarny, or the Kinyoun method or using the fluorescence auramine-rhodamine staining technique. In addition, polymerase chain reaction (PCR)-based detection techniques for various mycobacteria species can also be applied in both fresh and formalin-fixed paraffin-embedded tissues.[24]

T pallidum causing syphilis can involve the meninges and the spinal cord parenchyma as well as brain parenchyma. Approximately 5% of all patients with syphilis develop neural involvement in the form of meningitis or meningomyelitis.[25] Tabes dorsalis had been historically the most common presentation of in the spinal cord and is characterized by incoordination, pain, anesthesias, and visceral trophic abnormalities.[26] Before effective antibiotic treatment, Tabes dorsalis had been one of the more common presentations of neurosyphilis and seemed to be the only manifestation of neurosyphilis that was been markedly reduced during the antibiotic era.[27] Histologically, there is often inflammation within the leptomeninges and either atrophy or parenchymal destruction of the spinal cord. Tabes dorsalis is associated with demyelination of the posterior columns along with reactive gliosis. There is often thickening of the vessels, and meninges and the nerve tissue within the posterior nerve roots are often replaced by fibrosis and reactive changes. Meningomyelitis is often characterized by lymphoplasmacytic inflammation, dense fibrosis, and scattered granulomata with giant cells. Occasionally, there is clear necrotizing vasculitis with prominent perivascular inflammation.[9] A gumma is a well-circumscribed mass defined macroscopically and is a massive necrotizing granulomatous reaction composed of giant cells, epithelioid macrophages, and lymphoplasmacytic infiltrates. Gumma is most often localized to the meninges but can also involve the parenchyma. The dura is often markedly thickened near the gummae. Detection of Treponema species can be performed with the Dieterle stain, but the yield is not often satisfactory. Therefore, in suspected cases, serologic testing such as rapid plasma reagin and the antibody test (FTA-ABS [fluorescent treponemal antibody absorption]), immobilization reaction can be used to confirm the infectious agent. In recent years, PCR-based methods are preferred over standard serologic testing.[28]

B burgdorferi is the causative agent for Lyme disease and is transmitted often through ticks, most commonly in the northeastern United States, Wisconsin, and Michigan as well as the forested regions in California and Oregon. The clinical features can be quite variable, and their description is beyond the scope of this article; the reader is referred to more comprehensive review of the subject.[29,30] Typically, there is cerebrospinal fluid (CSF) pleocytosis with normal glucose and protein levels. CSF can be used for Western blot detection of antibodies or PCR detection of Borrelia DNA. Histologically, the spinal cord parenchyma and meninges can be affected and show lymphoplasmacytic infiltrates, microglial nodules, and astrocytosis. Nerve roots may show scarring, gliosis, and chronic inflammatory infiltrates. Nevertheless, spinal cord involvement in Lyme disease is extremely rare and may be in the form of acute transverse or posterior myelitis.[31,32] There is no useful special stain for the detection of borrelia in tissues, and serologic testing is not often specific, which necessitates detection by Western blotting.[33]

Other chronic infectious agents listed above often demonstrate nonspecific pathologic features, and their identification often relies on the level of suspicion for the agent and the availability of special stains, serologic, or molecular testing.

Mycoplasma pneumoniae is a common bacterial pathogen associated with respiratory infections and can occasionally cause infectious myelitis. Myelitis due to mycoplasma is extremely rare compared with infection in other sites and constitutes one of the most severe central nervous system (CNS) complications associated with this organism. In addition, many studies suggested an immune-mediated mechanism leading to acute transverse myelitis because of systemic mycoplasma infection or mycoplasma encephalitis.[34] Mycoplasma myelitis can have a wide range of clinical presentations, and the use of highly sensitive molecular diagnostic tests in the serum or the CSF may help to clearly define the cause. Histologic sampling (ie, an open biopsy) is often not needed and, when performed, typically demonstrates nonspecific inflammatory changes. Histologic diagnosis of mycoplasma is often not possible, and serologic methods have yielded variable results, making PCR-based detection the method of choice.[35,36]

Other bacterial myelitides include common and uncommon pathogens such as bartonella, rickettsiae, and chlamydia species.[37–39]

Fungal Infections

Although fungal infections involving the spinal cord or the meninges are rare, they have become more common in the HIV/AIDS era because of opportunistic agents such as *Candida*, *Aspergillus*, and *Zygomycetes*. Other fungal organisms such as *Cryptococcus, Coccidioides, Blastomyces*, and *Histoplasma* can primarily infect the spinal cord and cause myelitis or meningomyelitis as well as localized abscesses. Most of the organisms in this group, such as coccidioidomycosis, cryptococccosis, aspergillosis, and blastomycosis, cause granulomatous inflammation. In most fungal infections, there is CSF pleocytosis, and cultures and serologic studies from CSF are better initial attempts at identifying the organism before biopsy. In tissue samples, H&E stains may reveal the organisms such as *Candida* or *Aspergillus*, but others such as *Histoplasma* or *Cryptococci* may be elusive and require PAS stain or silver stains, such as Gomori methenamine silver (GMS) or immunohistochemistry. Most fungal organisms can be readily identified using special stains and will not require further analysis if appropriate tissue is obtained. For some fungal organisms, identification of the species using microbiological methods is indicated.

Aspergillus species often cause myelitis or meningomyelitis in the spinal cord through hematogenous spread and are typically angioinvasive, causing vasculitis or vascular occlusion.[40–43] Immune suppression such as HIV/AIDs, transplantation, or malignancies is a predisposing factor, and intracranial involvement with *Aspergillus* is equally prevalent.[40] Histologically, there is suppurative inflammation and often destruction of the vascular elastic lamina, vasculitis, and/or thrombosis. Abscess formation can be seen and typical granulomas form. The organism has septate hyphae that branch out in acute angles.

Cryptococci are encapsulated spherical yeast-like fungi causing granulomatous inflammation and are often associated with immune suppression. The fungus reaches the spinal cord hematogenous dissemination. Histologically, the fungi cause granulomatous inflammation and abscess formation particularly along the meninges.[44] The organism is a small, round, budding yeast surrounded by a thick capsule and is easily identified by GMS, India ink, mucicarmine, or PAS stains.

Coccidioides are endemic in semiarid regions in the world, such as southwestern United States and certain regions of the South American continent. Meningitis due to coccidioidomycosis is often in the setting of immune suppression leading to myelomeningitis and abscesses along the spinal cord.[45,46] The endospores are contained in large (20–60 μn) thick spherules that can be recognized on H&E stains; however, endospores are best identified on GMS and PAS stains. Inflammation is often accompanied by vasculitis and/or luminal occlusion of affected blood vessels. The granulomatous disease is often similar to tuberculous meningitis and abscess with well-formed granulomata containing the microorganisms.

Candida species are common throughout the world and are often opportunistic, causing significant pathologic abnormality in the setting of reduced immunity or immune suppression. The organisms the most common fungus associated with hospitalborne infections. Spinal and meningeal involvement often follows hematogenous dissemination, but they are distinctly rare and much less common than cerebral involvement.[47,48] Histologically, the organisms form pseudohyphae and true hyphae and are visible on H&E stains. However, most fungal stains such as GMS and PAS highlight both the pseudohyphae and the hyphae. The inflammation is often composed of microabscesses and acute and chronic inflammatory cells.

Histoplasma species are more common around river valleys, but are seen almost everywhere in the world, and the infection is often through inhalation. Dissemination and spinal involvement often occur in the setting of immune deficiency and often manifest as a meningeal inflammation.[49,50] The organism is rather small and is typically contained within the macrophages. Identification often requires special stains such as GMS and PAS. There is often a necrotizing chronic inflammation containing lymphocytes, plasma cells, macrophages, and giant cells.

Parasitic Infections

Myelitis and myelopathy can be caused by several parasitic organisms, but the incidence of such lesions is distinctly low. Typically, spinal cord involvement with parasitic infections is seen in tropical regions with poor sanitary conditions. However, with the increase of global travel and transactions, many such cases are also seen in the developed countries. *Echinococcus* species released from the canine tapeworm can cause spinal cysts or destructive paraspinal lesions leading to spinal cord compression; spinal involvement by cysticercosis caused by *Taenia solium* is seen in a minority of patients infected with this parasite in the tropics, but the brain is by far the most preferred site for cysticercosis. Finally, in patients with HIV/AIDS, toxoplasmosis can cause spinal abscesses and necrotizing myelitis. The reader is referred to more comprehensive reviews for a more detailed discussion of the parasitic infections of the CNS.[51] Identification of most parasitic infections usually requires well-sampled tissue and a simple H&E stain. Occasionally, such as in toxoplasmosis, identification may require immunohistochemical stains or serologic methods.

Viral Infections

Numerous viruses can involve the spinal cord and cause myelitis or myelopathy. Most often, viral organisms are associated with an acute myelitis, but many also cause a chronic infection that progresses like noninfectious chronic myelopathies. Viral myelitis can be either gray matter poliomyelitis or a white matter transverse/longitudinal myelitis. A comprehensive review of all the viruses associated with myelitis is beyond the scope of this article; however, some of the critical species associated with myelitis are mentioned.

Herpesviruses, HSV, varicella zoster virus (VZV), and CMV have been reported to cause significant myelitis.[52,53] VZV myelitis and typically radiculitis and myeloradiculitis have been well-recognized for a long time and are often the result of reactivation of the virus that remains latent within the dorsal ganglia as well as the sacral ganglia[54–56]; this occurs in individuals with diminished immune capacity or with frank immunosuppression, and the myelitis sometimes coexists with genital lesions. Histologic examination is often unnecessary, but rare samples obtained for other purposes demonstrate a variable amount of acute and chronic inflammatory cells with focal necrosis; intranuclear inclusions, known as Cowdry type A inclusions, are seen in glial, neuronal, and endothelial cells and can be detected serologically, histologically, or ultrastructurally. HSV-2 can cause radiculitis or myelitis in rare instances and is often accompanied by infection elsewhere. There may be coagulative necrosis of the spinal cord parenchyma and chronic inflammatory infiltrates within the leptomeninges, especially in immunosuppressed patients. Likewise, CMV has been known to cause transverse myelitis as a secondary site of involvement following primary infection.[57] Immunosuppression is the hallmark for all cases of myelitis caused by herpesviruses.

Enteroviruses, including polioviruses, cause myelitis, and until recently, polioviruses were the classic cause of acute flaccid paralysis. The virus had been nearly eradicated from the world because of an aggressive vaccination program by the World Health Organization (WHO).[58] Both inactivated (Salk) and active (Sabin) vaccines have been used effectively to virtually reduce the incidence to near zero.[59,60] However, several factors have prevented children in many countries from getting the vaccine.[61] Recently, based on the advice of the International Health Regulations Emergency Committee and its expert advisors, the WHO declared that the situation related to the international spread of wild poliovirus constitutes a Public Health Emergency of International Concern.[62] Histologically, poliovirus is associated with a low level of inflammatory infiltrate and loss of anterior neuron cells in the spinal cord. Other motor nuclei in the pons and medulla may also be affected. In the acute phase, there may be intense inflammation composed of neutrophils and lymphocytes, particularly involving the leptomeninges and the gray matter. The inflammation converts to a chronic inflammatory infiltrate composed of lymphocytes and macrophages with microscopic hemorrhages and neuronophagia. In the chronic phase, the inflammation subsides and there is loss of neurons, decrease of tissue, and atrophy in the anterior nerve roots. There are numerous enterovirus species that can present in atypical forms as aseptic meningitis, and molecular analyses in such cases may be necessary to identify the causative agent.[63]

Lentiviridae are a group of retroviruses (lenti for slow) that deliver RNA into the host cell and can have long incubation periods. These viruses also have the ability to infect nondividing cells. The HIV is the most notorious species in this family. HIV/AIDS is currently accepted as the term that represents the entire range of pathologic processes and the clinical manifestation of HIV infection in humans. Transmission is typically via contact with contaminated blood, sexual intercourse, pregnancy, and transfusions. Spinal cord disease associated with HIV infection includes a long list of secondary pathogens in addition to direct infection by the virus.[9] HIV-associated vacuolar myelopathy had been one of the most common spinal cord pathologic abnormalities during the HIV/AIDS epidemic.[64–66] Vacuolar myelopathy has been assumed to occur in the setting of advanced immunosuppression, and the incidence has declined with the use of effective multiple drug regimens. The histologic features of HIV-associated vacuolar myelopathy are often characterized by loss of myelin and spongy degeneration involving the lateral and posterior columns.[67] The white matter has a vacuolar appearance with scattered macrophages and rare lymphocytic cells. Inflammation is typically very sparse and rare perivascular multinucleated giant cells can be seen. Because there is no correlation between the severity and location of vacular myelopathy with the HIV burden, mechanisms other than direct viral cytopathic effect have been suggested.[65]

Box 1
Histologic patterns of infections in the spinal cord

- Acute necrotizing myelitis/meningomyelitis: Presence of polymorphonuclear leukocytes with necrosis along Virchow-Robin spaces, with or without parenchymal inflammation
  - Group B streptococci
  - *L monocytogenes*
  - *E coli*
  - *S pneumoniae*
  - *N meningitidis*
  - *H influenza*
  - *Aspergillus* species
  - *Candida* species
  - Other, uncommon pathogens
- Chronic lymphocytic meningitis: Lymphocytic and plasma cell inflammation predominantly involving the leptomeninges and Virchow-Robin spaces. May also include scattered eosinophilic infiltrate
  - *Enterovirus* species
  - Herpesviridae (HSV, VZV, CMV)
  - Lentiviridae (HIV, human T-lymphotropic virus-1)
- Acute necrotizing myelitis with or without Abscess formation: Predominantly polymorphonuclear leukocytes with destructive necrosis involving the parenchyma and Virchow-Robin spaces with or without collection of pus and cavity formation
  - Bacterial infections causing acute necrotizing meningitis (see above)
  - *Mycobacteriae* (tuberculosis, leprosy)
  - *Treponema* species (syphilis)
  - *Actinomycetes* species
  - *Nocardia* species
  - *Aspergillosis* species
  - *Coccidioidomycetes*
  - *Candida* species
  - Toxoplasma
  - Entameoba and Balamuthia
- Chronic myelitis: Parenchymal lymphocytic and plasmacytic infiltrates with microglial nodules, occasional neuronophagia, and macrophage infiltrate without granuloma formation
  - Progressive multifocal leukoencephalopathy (JC virus)
  - Herpesviridae (HSV-chronic, CMV)
  - Lentiviridae (HIV)
  - *Leptospira* species
  - *Borreliosis* (Lyme disease)
- Granulomatous meningomyelitis: Granulomata composed of lymphoplasmacytic infiltrates surrounding epithelioid histiocytes and giant cells with or without a necrotic core
  - *Mycobacteriae* (tuberculosis, leprosy)
  - *Treponema* (syphilis)
  - *Tropheryma* (Whipple disease)
  - *Aspergillus* species
  - *Cryptococcus* species
  - *Blastomycetes* species
  - *Histoplasma* species
  - Enteameoba and Balamuthia

Detection of viral infections can rarely be done using light microscopic stains and often require ultrastructural analysis of the tissue using electron microscopy (EM). Analysis of tissues using EM requires special fixation and processing, so tissue must be specifically submitted for ultrastructural evaluation. In many cases, sampling of the tissue is critical in correct identification. Recently, more effective and faster techniques using either single-probe or multiplex PCR-based techniques have been quite successful in the identification of viral pathogens.[68] These techniques not only are effective for the diagnosis of common viruses but also greatly improve the ability to detect emerging viral infections.[69] Recent studies using next-generation sequencing seem quite promising in the identification of elusive pathogens.[70]

SPONDYLITIS AND DISCIITIS

Although this article predominantly provides a review of the primary infections of the medulla spinalis and its dura, more prevalent and troublesome infections involve the intervertabral disc (discitis) and/or the vertebrae (spondylitis) with or without the involvement of the joint space (spondylarthritis). Infectious spine disease is much less common than degenerative spine or disc disease, but it can still be a significant health problem in many countries.[71] Many conditions such as chronic debilitating disease in the elderly, malignancies, diabetes, surgical manipulations of the spine or the disc, intravenous drug abuse, and emerging infections like tuberculosis may lead to an increased incidence of infectious spondylitis or discitis. Tuberculous spondylitis is more frequent in the developing world and in areas with limited access to health care. Tuberculous spondylitis may have unusual clinical and radiological presentations, especially in the setting of HIV/AIDS.[72] In certain partsof the world, however, pyogenic spondylodiscitis seems to be more frequent than tuberculous spondylodiscitis.[71] Hematological parameters as well as the histologic features and microbiological cultures can easily distinguish between pyogenic and tuberculous spondylodiscitis quite easily.

In terms of location, lumbar vertebrae seem to be more commonly affected by infectious spondylodiscitis, especially by pyogenic infections, and some suggest that tuberculous spondylodiscitis is more common in the thoracic vertebrae. Radioimaging-guided biopsies for the diagnoses of the microorganism in infectious spondylitis have often high yields, if the diagnostic procedure is performed in cooperation with the pathologists to confirm the adequacy of the specimen. In recent studies, the most common infectious agents were identified as mycobacterium tuberculosis and gram-positive bacteria.[73]

Although radiological studies provide critical information, a review of the clinical and radiological features of infectious spondylitis is beyond the scope of this article, and the reader is referred to more comprehensive reviews in this subject.[74] In addition, to common bacterial infections, fungal and parasitic agents can also be encountered as causative agents of infectious spondylitis, particularly in the immune-compromised patient. Pathologic assessment in such cases along with the special studies mentioned above often provides the specific diagnosis in most patients. Communication between the surgical team and the pathologist and exchange of specific information on the patient's clinical and radiological features are critical for selection and performance of appropriate histologic analysis that will facilitate the diagnosis. In atypical presentations or radiological features, early involvement of the pathologist during the radioimaging-guided biopsies or intraoperative frozen sections will greatly enhance this selection of appropriate workup of the pathologic specimen (**Boxes 1** and **2**).

Box 2
What the referring physician needs to know

- It is critical to recognize the clinical and radiological pattern of the spinal infectious process to enable a differential diagnosis of infections before obtaining any tissue for pathologic and microbiological assessment.

- Pathologic and microbiological assessment of any infection should be performed in coordination to gather the most comprehensive information and accurate identification of the pathogen.

- It is critical to select the appropriate biological sample at the appropriate time for pathogen identification, and the referring physician should be familiar with the best method of identification for the pathogen in question.

- Direct communication with the pathologist and the microbiologist before taking a definitive action often avoids missed opportunities for the correct identification of the disease.

REFERENCES

1. West TW, Hess C, Cree BA. Acute transverse myelitis: demyelinating, inflammatory, and infectious myelopathies. Semin Neurol 2012;32(2):97–113.

2. Richie MB, Pruitt AA. Spinal cord infections. Neurol Clin 2013;31(1):19–53.

3. Mihai C, Jubelt B. Infectious myelitis. Curr Neurol Neurosci Rep 2012;12(6):633–41.

4. Bleck TP. Bacterial meningitis and other nonviral infections of the nervous system. Crit Care Clin 2013; 29(4):975–87.

5. Morris BJ, Fletcher N, Davis RA, et al. Bacterial meningitis after traumatic thoracic fracture-dislocation: two case reports and review of the literature. J Orthop Trauma 2010;24(5):e49–53.

6. Bhattacharya M, Joshi N. Spinal epidural abscess with myelitis and meningitis caused by Streptococcus pneumoniae in a young child. J Spinal Cord Med 2011;34(3):340–3.

7. Steinlin M, Knecht B, Konu D, et al. Neonatal Escherichia coli meningitis: spinal adhesions as a late complication. Eur J Pediatr 1999;158(12):968–70.

8. Baumann M, Birnbacher R, Koch J, et al. Uncommon manifestations of neuroborreliosis in children. Eur J Paediatr Neurol 2010;14(3):274–7.

9. Berger JR. Infectious myelopathies. Continuum (Minneap Minn) 2011;17(4):761–75.

10. Kristopaitis T, Jensen R, Gujrati M. Clostridium perfringens: a rare cause of postoperative spinal surgery meningitis. Surg Neurol 1999;51(4):448–50 [discussion: 450–1].

11. Marshman LA, Hardwidge C, Donaldson PM. Bacillus cereus meningitis complicating cerebrospinal fluid fistula repair and spinal drainage. Br J Neurosurg 2000;14(6):580–2.

12. Newton JA Jr, Lesnik IK, Kennedy CA. Streptococcus salivarius meningitis following spinal anesthesia. Clin Infect Dis 1994;18(5):840–1.

13. Almeida N, Portela F, Oliveira P, et al. Meningitis in a patient with previously undiagnosed Crohn's disease. Inflamm Bowel Dis 2009;15(5):643–5.

14. Maggiore R, Miller F, Stryker S, et al. Meningitis and epidural abscess associated with fistulizing Crohn's disease. Dig Dis Sci 2004;49(9):1461–5.

15. Helbok R, Broessner G, Pfausler B, et al. Chronic meningitis. J Neurol 2009;256(2):168–75.

16. Gall D, Nielsen K, Nicola A, et al. A proficiency testing method for detecting antibodies against Brucella abortus in quantitative and qualitative serological tests. Rev Sci Tech 2008;27(3):819–28.

17. Byun SK, Jung SC, Yoo HS. Random amplification of polymorphic DNA typing of Listeria monocytogenes isolated from meat. Int J Food Microbiol 2001;69(3): 227–35.

18. Shim WB, Choi JG, Kim JY, et al. Enhanced rapidity for qualitative detection of Listeria monocytogenes using an enzyme-linked immunosorbent assay and immunochromatography strip test combined with immunomagnetic bead separation. J Food Prot 2008;71(4):781–9.

19. Lindblom A, Severinson K, Nilsson K. Rickettsia felis infection in Sweden: report of two cases with subacute meningitis and review of the literature. Scand J Infect Dis 2010;42(11–12):906–9.

20. Jenkins HE, Tolman AW, Yuen CM, et al. Incidence of multidrug-resistant tuberculosis disease in children: systematic review and global estimates. Lancet 2014;383(9928):1572–9.

21. Gropper MR, Schulder M, Sharan AD, et al. Central nervous system tuberculosis: medical management and surgical indications. Surg Neurol 1995; 44:378–85.

22. Pellise F. Tuberculosis and Pott's disease, still very relevant health problems. Eur Spine J 2013; 22(Suppl 4):527–8.

23. Malhotra HS. Diagnostic imaging in Pott's disease of the spine. N Am J Med Sci 2013;5(7):412–3.

24. Anilkumar AK, Madhavilatha GK, Paul LK, et al. Standardization and evaluation of a tetraplex polymerase chain reaction to detect and differentiate Mycobacterium tuberculosis complex and nontuberculous Mycobacteria–a retrospective study on pulmonary TB patients. Diagn Microbiol Infect Dis 2012;72(3): 239–47.

25. Berger JR, Dean D. Neurosyphilis. Handb Clin Neurol 2014;121:1461–72.

26. Chilver-Stainer L, Fischer U, Hauf M, et al. Syphilitic myelitis: rare, nonspecific, but treatable. Neurology 2009;72(7):673–5.

27. Timmermans M, Carr J. Neurosyphilis in the modern era. J Neurol Neurosurg Psychiatry 2004;75(12): 1727–30.

28. Leslie DE, Azzato F, Karapanagiotidis T, et al. Development of a real-time PCR assay to detect Treponema pallidum in clinical specimens and assessment of the assay's performance by comparison with serological testing. J Clin Microbiol 2007;45(1):93–6.

29. Logigian EL, Kaplan RF, Steere AC. Chronic neurologic manifestations of Lyme disease. N Engl J Med 1990;323:1438–44.

30. Fernandez RE, Rothberg M, Ferencz G, et al. Lyme disease of the CNS: MR imaging findings in 14 cases. AJNR Am J Neuroradiol 1990;11:479–81.

31. Halperin JJ. Nervous system Lyme disease. Handb Clin Neurol 2014;121:1473–83.

32. Blanc F, Froelich S, Vuillemet F, et al. Acute myelitis and Lyme disease. Rev Neurol (Paris) 2007;163(11): 1039–47 [in French].

33. Tylewska-Wierzbanowska S, Chmielewski T. Limitation of serological testing for Lyme borreliosis: evaluation of ELISA and western blot in comparison with PCR and culture methods. Wien Klin Wochenschr 2002;114(13–14):601–5.

34. Tsiodras S, Kelesidis T, Kelesidis I, et al. Mycoplasma pneumoniae-associated myelitis: a comprehensive review. Eur J Neurol 2006;13(2):112–24.

35. Qu J, Gu L, Wu J, et al. Accuracy of IgM antibody testing, FQ-PCR and culture in laboratory diagnosis of acute infection by Mycoplasma pneumoniae in

adults and adolescents with community-acquired pneumonia. BMC Infect Dis 2013;13:172.

36. Waites KB. What's new in diagnostic testing and treatment approaches for Mycoplasma pneumoniae infections in children? Adv Exp Med Biol 2011;719: 47–57.

37. Lee KL, Lee JK, Yim YM, et al. Acute transverse myelitis associated with scrub typhus: case report and a review of literatures. Diagn Microbiol Infect Dis 2008;60(2):237–9.

38. Crook T, Bannister B. Acute transverse myelitis associated with Chlamydia psittaci infection. J Infect 1996;32(2):151–2.

39. Baylor P, Garoufi A, Karpathios T, et al. Transverse myelitis in 2 patients with Bartonella henselae infection (cat scratch disease). Clin Infect Dis 2007; 45(4):e42–5.

40. Boes B, Bashir R, Boes C, et al. Central nervous system aspergillosis. Analysis of 26 patients. J Neuroimaging 1994;4(3):123–9.

41. Mollahoseini R, Nikoobakht M. Diffuse myelitis after treatment of cerebral aspergillosis in an immune competent patient. Acta Med Iran 2011;49(6):402–6.

42. Rodrigo N, Perera KN, Ranwala R, et al. Aspergillus meningitis following spinal anaesthesia for caesarean section in Colombo, Sri Lanka. Int J Obstet Anesth 2007;16(3):256–60.

43. Yanai Y, Wakao T, Fukamachi A, et al. Intracranial granuloma caused by aspergillus fumigatus. Surg Neurol 1985;23:597–604.

44. Shen CC, Cheng WY, Yang MY. Isolated intramedullary cryptococcal granuloma of the conus medullaris: case report and review of the literature. Scand J Infect Dis 2006;38(6–7):562–5.

45. Elgafy H, Miller J, Meyers S, et al. Disseminated coccidioidomycosis of the spine in an immunocompetent patient. Am J Orthop (Belle Mead NJ) 2014; 43(8):E181–4.

46. Lammering JC, Iv M, Gupta N, et al. Imaging spectrum of CNS coccidioidomycosis: prevalence and significance of concurrent brain and spinal disease. AJR Am J Roentgenol 2013;200(6):1334–46.

47. Goldani LZ, Santos RP. Candida tropicalis as an emerging pathogen in Candida meningitis: case report and review. Braz J Infect Dis 2010;14(6): 631–3.

48. Sakayama K, Kidani T, Matsuda Y, et al. Subdural spinal granuloma resulting from Candida albicans without immunosufficiency: case report. Spine (Phila Pa 1976) 2002;27(15):E356–60.

49. Wheat LJ, Batteiger BE, Sathapatayavongs B. Histoplasma capsulatum infections of the central nervous system. A clinical review. Medicine (Baltimore) 1990; 69(4):244–60.

50. Voelker JL, Muller J, Worth RM. Intramedullary spinal Histoplasma granuloma. Case report. J Neurosurg 1989;70(6):959–61.

51. Finsterer J, Auer H. Parasitoses of the human central nervous system. J Helminthol 2013;87(3):257–70.

52. Irani DN. Aseptic meningitis and viral myelitis. Neurol Clin 2008;26(3):635–55, vii–viii.

53. Whitley RJ. Herpes simplex virus infections of the central nervous system. A review. Am J Med 1988; 85(Suppl 2A):61–6.

54. Gray F, Bélec L, Lescs MC, et al. Varicella-zoster virus infection of the central nervous system in the acquired immune dificiency syndrome. Brain 1994; 117:987–99.

55. Schmidbauer M, Budka H, Pilz P, et al. Presence, distribution and spread of productive varicella zoster virus infection in nervous tissues. Brain 1992; 115:383–98.

56. Gilden DH, Vafai A, Shtram Y, et al. Varicella-zoster virus DNA in human sensory ganglia. Nature 1983; 306(5942):478–80.

57. Fux CA, Pfister S, Nohl F, et al. Cytomegalovirus-associated acute transverse myelitis in immunocompetent adults. Clin Microbiol Infect 2003;9(12): 1187–90.

58. Willyard C. Polio: the eradication endgame. Nature 2014;507(7490):S14–5.

59. Polio vaccines: WHO position paper, January 2014. Wkly Epidemiol Rec 2014;89(9):73–92.

60. Progress towards polio eradication worldwide, 2013-2014. Wkly Epidemiol Rec 2014;89(22):237–44.

61. Polio has not gone away. Arch Dis Child 2014; 99(2):170.

62. Eurosurveillance Editorial Team. Note from the editors: WHO declares international spread of wild poliovirus a public health emergency of international concern. Euro Surveill 2014;19(18).

63. Valcour V, Haman A, Cornes S, et al. A case of enteroviral meningoencephalitis presenting as rapidly progressive dementia. Nat Clin Pract Neurol 2008;4(7):399–403.

64. Dal Pan GJ, Glass JD, McArthur JC. Clinicopathologic correlations of HIV-1-associated vacuolar myelopathy: an autopsy-based case-control study. Neurology 1994;44(11):2159–64.

65. Di Rocco A, Werner P. Hypothesis on the pathogenesis of vacuolar myelopathy, dementia, and peripheral neuropathy in AIDS. J Neurol Neurosurg Psychiatry 1999;66(4):554.

66. Sartoretti-Schefer S, Blattler T, Wichmann W. Spinal MRI in vacuolar myelopathy, and correlation with histopathological findings. Neuroradiology 1997; 39(12):865–9.

67. Petito CK, Navia BA, Cho ES, et al. Vacuolar myelopathy pathologically resembling subacute combined degeneration in patients with the acquired immunodeficiency syndrome. N Engl J Med 1985;312(14):874–9.

68. Wang D, Urisman A, Liu YT, et al. Viral discovery and sequence recovery using DNA microarrays. PLoS Biol 2003;1(2):E2.

69. Wilson MR. Emerging viral infections. Curr Opin Neurol 2013;26(3):301–6.

70. Wilson MR, Naccache SN, Samayoa E, et al. Actionable diagnosis of neuroleptospirosis by next-generation sequencing. N Engl J Med 2014; 370(25):2408–17.

71. Jeong SJ, Choi SW, Youm JY, et al. Microbiology and epidemiology of infectious spinal disease. J Korean Neurosurg Soc 2014;56(1):21–7.

72. Danaviah S, Govender S, Cassol S. Histopathology and genotyping in infectious spondylitis of HIV- and HIV+ patients. Clin Orthop Relat Res 2007; 460:50–5.

73. Kim BJ, Lee JW, Kim SJ, et al. Diagnostic yield of fluoroscopy-guided biopsy for infectious spondylitis. AJNR Am J Neuroradiol 2013;34(1):233–8.

74. Forrester DM. Infectious spondylitis. Semin Ultrasound CT MR 2004;25(6):461–73.

Pediatric Spinal Infection and Inflammation

Andrea Rossi, MD

KEYWORDS

- Pediatrics • Spine • Inflammation • Infection

KEY POINTS

- Inflammatory and infectious disorders of the spine in children are less common than in adults, and are usually categorized according to location into (1) those predominantly affecting the spinal cord; (2) those predominantly affecting the nerve roots and meninges; and (3) those predominantly affecting the vertebrae, discs, and epidural space.
- Magnetic resonance (MR) imaging is the main imaging modality for diagnosing infectious and inflammatory disorders of the spine in the pediatric age group.
- Because of the often aspecific clinical presentation that may raise the suspicion of spinal cord compression, MR imaging is often performed in emergencies.
- Intravenous administration of contrast material (ie, gadolinium chelate) is of paramount importance for an adequate identification and characterization of these disorders.

INTRODUCTION

Inflammatory and infectious disorders of the spine in children are less common than in adults, and are usually categorized according to location into (1) those predominantly affecting the spinal cord; (2) those predominantly affecting the nerve roots and meninges; and (3) those predominantly affecting the vertebrae, discs, and epidural space.

DISORDERS PREDOMINANTLY AFFECTING THE SPINAL CORD

Disorders primitively involving the spinal cord may be grouped into 2 basic categories: (1) inflammatory disorders, represented by acute transverse myelopathy; and (2) infectious disorders, which may be bacterial, viral, fungal, or parasitic. Inflammatory spinal cord diseases are much more common than primitive spinal cord infection.

Acute Transverse Myelopathy

Acute transverse myelopathy (ATM) is a focal inflammatory disorder of the spinal cord resulting in motor, sensory, and autonomic dysfunction. Individuals of all ages may be affected, with bimodal peaks between the ages of 10 and 19 years and 30 and 39 years. Although the terms ATM and acute transverse myelitis have often been used interchangeably, the former is a broad header that includes idiopathic forms (corresponding with acute transverse myelitis) and forms with known cause, such as postinfectious/postvaccination (ie, acute disseminated encephalomyelitis [ADEM]); neuromyelitis optica; multiple sclerosis; and ischemic, paraneoplastic, autoimmune, and postirradiation myelitis.

Idiopathic Acute Transverse Myelopathy

Clinical presentation is with pain, paresthesias, leg weakness, and sphincteral dysfunction, all of which progress to nadir between 4 hours and 21 days (usually 24 hours) following the onset of symptoms. It is thought that strokelike evolution (ie, nadir reached earlier than 4 hours) indicates vascular causes (spinal cord infarction). Signs and/or symptoms are usually bilateral, although not necessarily symmetric, and there usually is a

Disclosure: None.
Department of Pediatric Neuroradiology, Istituto Giannina Gaslini, Via G. Gaslini 5, Genova I-16147, Italy
E-mail address: andrearossi@ospedale-gaslini.ge.it

Neuroimag Clin N Am 25 (2015) 173–191
http://dx.doi.org/10.1016/j.nic.2015.01.001

clearly defined sensory level. Cerebrospinal fluid (CSF) analysis reveals signs of spinal cord inflammation, such as pleocytosis or increased immunoglobulin G (IgG) index.

The diagnosis of idiopathic ATM is one of exclusion, and involves 3 consecutive steps[1]:

1. Rule out a compressive cause: this requires contrast-enhanced magnetic resonance (MR) imaging of the entire spinal cord; if cord compression is ruled out and MR imaging indicates primary spinal cord involvement, MR imaging of the brain should also be performed;
2. Define presence or absence of spinal cord inflammation by performing lumbar puncture with CSF analysis;
3. Define extent of demyelination: brain MR imaging is analyzed for signs of involvement of the white matter and optic nerves. If none

is found, idiopathic ATM is likely. If the white matter is involved, ADEM or multiple sclerosis should be considered. In addition, if the optic nerves are the only involved structure, neuromyelitis optica is likely. Visual evoked potentials are a significant diagnostic adjunct.

MR imaging criteria for myelitis (Fig. 1)[2,3] include normal or slightly expanded spinal cord showing diffuse or patchy hyperintensity on T2-weighted images, usually involving more than 1 vertebral level in length. There may be patchy enhancement after gadolinium administration. The conus medullaris is involved most frequently.

Prognosis of idiopathic ATM is variable, with one-third of patients recovering with little to no sequelae, one-third left with moderate degrees of permanent disability, and one-third having severe disabilities.[1] Rapid progression of signs and

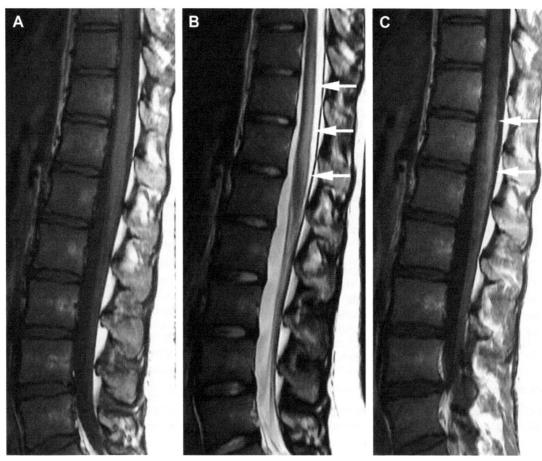

Fig. 1. Idiopathic acute transverse myelitis in a 14-year-old girl. (*A*) Sagittal T1-weighted image, (*B*) sagittal T2-weighted image, (*C*) Gd-enhanced sagittal T1-weighted image, (*D, E*) axial T2-weighted images, and (*F, G*) Gd-enhanced axial T1-weighted images. There is a slightly swollen lower thoracic cord and conus medullaris showing hyperintensity on T2-weighted images (*arrows, B, D, E*) and mild contrast enhancement (*arrows, C, F, G*). Signal abnormalities prevail in the posterior portion of the cord in this case.

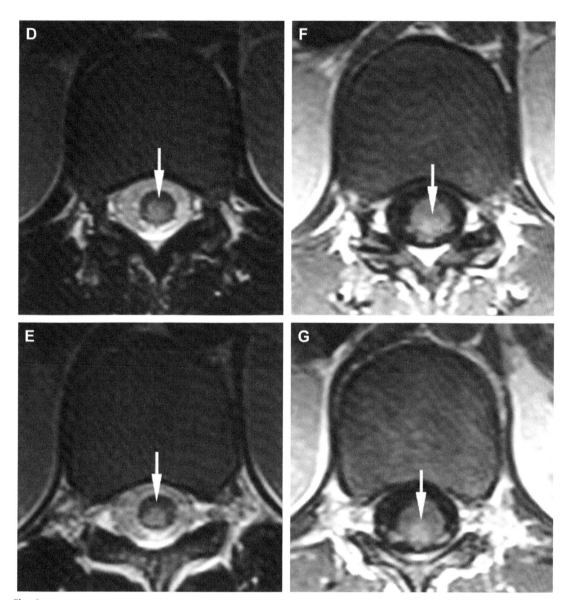

Fig. 1.

symptoms at presentation usually portends a poor prognosis.

Acute Disseminated Encephalomyelitis

ADEM has been associated with viral infections (ie, postinfectious myelitis), such as measles, rubella, chickenpox, mumps, influenza, Epstein-Barr virus, Coxsackie B, cytomegalovirus, herpes simplex virus, hepatitis A virus, and adenoviruses, as well as with Borrelia, Mycoplasma pneumoniae, and nonspecific infection of the upper respiratory tract. Moreover, ADEM may also occur after vaccination (ie, postvaccination myelitis), including polio, rabies, smallpox, influenza, rubella, and plasma-derived

form of hepatitis B.[4] In most patients, postvaccination myelitis is a presumptive diagnosis based on the temporal relationship between vaccine administration and onset of symptoms.

Unlike idiopathic ATM, ADEM typically is characterized by extensive involvement of the brain. About 40% of patients with ADEM also show lesions in their spinal cords.[5] The process usually is monophasic (ie, it occurs once in the life of the patient). However, multifocal disseminated encephalomyelitis has also been documented.[6]

The disorder commonly begins 1 to 2 weeks after a viral, and seemingly minor, illness. The initial illness is often subclinical. Once the symptoms are present, they become more obvious 1 to

2 days after the diagnosis but may progress for up to 2 weeks. CSF analysis may show increased proteins and leukocytosis. The thoracic spinal cord is involved more often than the cervical region. On histology, there is necrosis and inflammation; perivascular lymphocytic infiltration and demyelination also are present.

On MR imaging, T2-weighted images may show multiple, more or less well-defined areas of increased signal intensity within the cord (Fig. 2).[7] Holocord involvement is possible. Segmental disease generally involves 2 to 3 vertebral bodies in length, and may expand the cord slightly. In ADEM, generally there is no enhancement after gadolinium administration, whereas enhancement is common in idiopathic ATM.[2] In the latter condition, enhancement of the cauda equina may also be seen, suggesting that

transverse myelitis and Guillain-Barré syndrome (GBS) may have a similar cause.

Multiple Sclerosis

Multiple sclerosis (MS) is rare in children, and spinal cord involvement is even rarer. Spinal cord plaques occur preferentially in the dorsolateral cord, and may be found at any segment.[8,9] A predilection for the cervical segment has been reported in the early stages of the disease.[9]

The MR imaging findings in childhood and juvenile MS mimic those of adult-onset MS.[10] T2-weighted images show 1 or more elongated, poorly marginated, hyperintense intramedullary lesions. Acute demyelinating lesions may display mass effect and enhance after gadolinium administration (Fig. 3).[9]

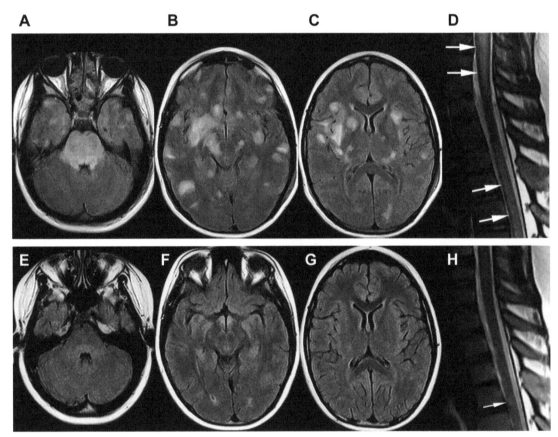

Fig. 2. Acute disseminated encephalomyelitis in a 14-year-old boy with prior upper respiratory infection: findings at presentation and follow-up. (A–C) Axial fluid-attenuated inversion recovery (FLAIR) images and (D) sagittal T2-weighted image at presentation. There are multiple hyperintense areas that involve both the gray and white matter of the brain asymmetrically (A–C); note the marked swelling of the pons (A). There also are hyperintense lesions involving the spinal cord at various locations (arrows, D). (E–G) Axial FLAIR images and (H) sagittal T2-weighted image at 3 months' follow-up. Brain findings are now back to normal (E–G). There is some residual hyperintensity of the spinal cord (arrow, H).

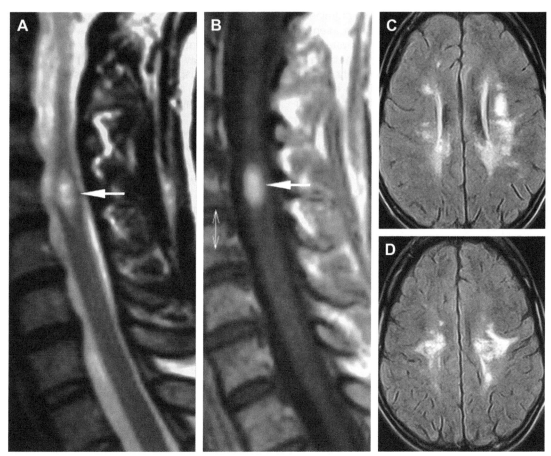

Fig. 3. MS in a 15-year-old girl. (A) Sagittal T2-weighted image, (B) Gd-enhanced sagittal T1-weighted image, and (C, D) axial FLAIR images. There is a T2 hyperintense lesion that causes slight cord swelling at C4 level (arrow, A). The lesion enhances markedly with gadolinium (arrow, B). Note the multiple brain plaques in a typical distribution (C, D).

Tumefactive plaques in the spinal cord have been reported in association with swelling and MR signal changes mimicking a neoplasm.[11]

Neuromyelitis Optica

Neuromyelitis optica (NMO), formerly known as Devic disease, is a rare, severe, monophasic or multiphasic demyelinating disease of the central nervous system (CNS) that preferentially affects the optic nerves and spinal cord. The revised diagnostic criteria for NMO[12] require the presence of optic neuritis and acute myelitis, associated with either a spinal MR imaging lesion extending over 3 or more segments, or positive NMO serology. It has been shown that presence of at least 2 of the following 3 laboratory findings is 99% sensitive and 90% specific for NMO: (1) contiguous spinal cord MR imaging lesion extending over more than 3 vertebral segments, (2) brain MR imaging not meeting criteria for MS, and (3) NMO-IgG seropositive status.[13] NMO-IgG is an autoantibody found in the serum of patients affected by NMO, with 91% to 100% specificity and 75% to 90% sensitivity. NMO-IgG binds to aquaporin-4 (AQP4), which is the main channel that regulates water homeostasis in the CNS, mainly located around cerebral microvessels, pia mater, and Virchow-Robin sheaths.

Most affected patients are female, with a 9:1 gender predilection compared with male patients.[13] Although mostly a disease of adults, NMO occasionally is seen in children. Typically, optic neuritis is severe, painful, unilateral rather than bilateral, and not simultaneous with ATM. Attacks of optic neuritis precede ATM in 80% of cases (usually <3 months), whereas ATM precedes optic neuritis in 20% of cases. Clinical findings in patients with myelitis prominently include severe symmetric paraplegia, sensory loss below the lesion, and bladder dysfunction. Atypical forms of NMO have recently been identified in which NMO-IgG seropositivity is found in patients with isolated longitudinally extensive transverse myelitis (LETM), monophasic or recurrent isolated optic neuritis, and brainstem encephalitis.[14] The terms NMO spectrum disorder and autoimmune AQP4 channelopathy describe this host of conditions that encompass a larger group of patients than the classic NMO criteria.[15]

Imaging of the entire craniospinal axis should always be performed in patients suspected of having NMO.[15] Spinal MR imaging (Fig. 4) typically shows LETM, characterized by large, confluent areas of high T2 signal intensity involving the spinal cord extensively.[16] These lesions are typically longer than 3 vertebral bodies in a craniocaudal direction; they occasionally involve the entire span of the cord, and may enhance with gadolinium administration.[15] The cord may be expanded and may show cavitation. Brain imaging of patients with suspected NMO shows optic nerve and chiasm involvement, characterized by swelling, T2-hyperintensity, and contrast enhancement in the acute demyelination phase. Although the brain may be unaffected, hypothalamic, periaqueductal gray, and area postrema lesions can be found in the context of NMO in up to 60% of cases in some studies.[15]

SPINAL CORD INFECTIONS
Spinal Cord Abscess/Granuloma

Bacterial spinal cord abscesses are extremely rare.[17] Children account for up 20% to 50% of cases in some series. Among causative

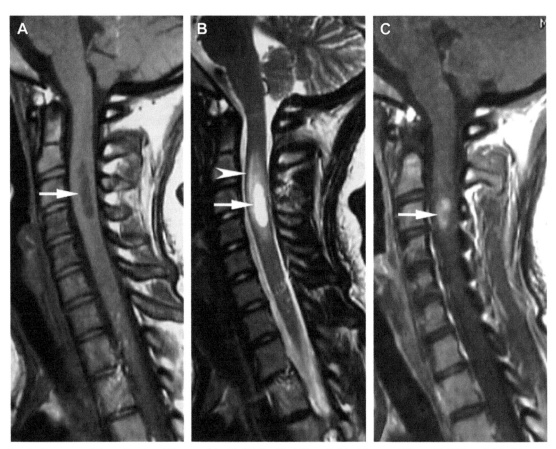

Fig. 4. Neuromyelitis optica in a 16-year-old girl. (*A*) Sagittal T1-weighted image, (*B*) sagittal T2-weighted image, and (*C*) Gd-enhanced sagittal T1-weighted image obtained 1 month after an episode of optic neuritis and during an episode of acute transverse myelitis. The cervical cord is slightly swollen and shows a central cavitation (*arrows, A, B*) at the C3-4 level, surrounded by edema (*arrowhead, B*). Slightly off-midline enhancing focus is seen after gadolinium (*arrow, C*).

organisms, *Schistosoma* is particularly common in children. Tuberculosis is also gaining new ground in Western countries. Fungal diseases include candida infection, aspergillus, and nocardiosis. Predisposing conditions include congenital heart disease, disorders of the immune system, patients with long-term intravascular access lines, underlying spinal cord tumors, and dermal sinuses. Dermal sinuses may give rise to intraspinal abscesses outside and inside the spinal cord.[18] Most patients have a history of infection elsewhere and spinal cord involvement may be secondary to either hematogenous or lymphatic spread. The process begins as a myelitis and, if left untreated, may progress to frank abscess formation.

MR imaging shows increased T2 signal intensity and expansion of the cord. A thin hypointense stripe surrounding the lesion indicates a capsule. After contrast administration there is ill-defined or well-defined marginal enhancement according to the stage of the inflammatory process (**Figs. 5** and **6**).[17] After initiation of treatment, the signal on T2-weighted images decreases and ring enhancement becomes prominent. With adequate therapy, the enhancement slowly resolves.

Viral Myelitis

Viral myelitis may be caused by poliovirus, herpes zoster infection, and cytomegalovirus, especially associated with acquired immunodeficiency syndrome. Although poliomyelitis is now uncommon,[19] myelitis secondary to herpes zoster infection occurs more frequently.[20] The symptoms and MR imaging findings generally correspond closely with the dermatomal distribution of the lesions. The presence of a sensory abnormality accompanied by the characteristic vesicular rash should make clinicians suspect a herpes zoster myelitis. On T2-weighted images, the spinal cord shows a focal, rounded, hyperintense lesion involving one-half of the cord ipsilateral to the cutaneous rash. Contrast enhancement may occur (**Fig. 7**). It is not clear whether the myelitis is caused by an allergic reaction, autoimmune

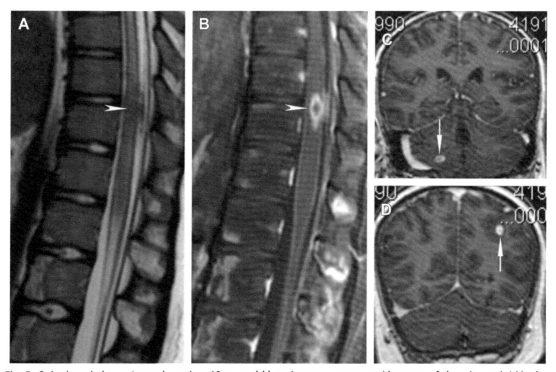

Fig. 5. Spinal cord abscess/granuloma in a 10-year-old boy, immunosuppressed because of chronic myeloid leukemia. (*A*) Sagittal T2-weighted image, (*B*) Gd-enhanced fat-suppressed sagittal T1-weighted image, and (*C, D*) Gd-enhanced coronal T1-weighted images. There is a small intramedullary lesion showing a tiny hypointense periphery on T2-weighted images (*arrowhead, A*) and a strongly enhancing capsule (*arrowhead, B*). Brain imaging shows additional ring-enhancing lesions in the right cerebellar hemisphere (*arrow, C*) and left parietal lobe (*arrow, D*). Candidosis was eventually diagnosed. (*Courtesy of* M. Thurnher, MD, Vienna, Austria.)

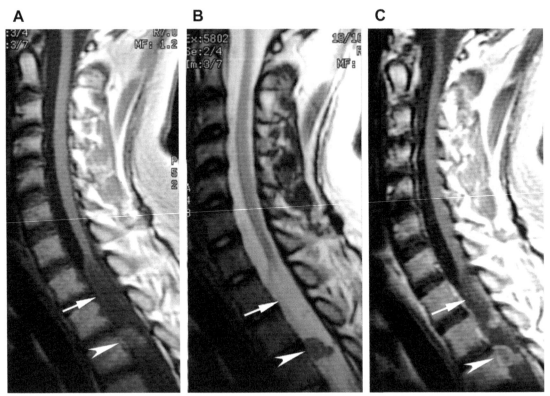

Fig. 6. Tubercular myelitis and granulomas. (*A*) Sagittal T1-weighted image, (*B*) sagittal T2-weighted image, and (*C*) Gd-enhanced sagittal T1-weighted image. In this patient with known tuberculosis, there is marked swelling of the thoracic cord showing increased T1 and T2 relaxation times (*arrow, A–C*). Discrete intramedullary nodular lesions show higher T1 signal, lower T2 signal, and ringlike enhancement (*arrowhead, A–C*). (*Courtesy of* T. Tali, MD, Ankara, Turkey.)

vasculitis, demyelination, or by direct viral infection. Viruses are generally absent in the CSF.

DISORDERS PREDOMINANTLY AFFECTING THE NERVE ROOTS AND MENINGES
Bacterial Meningitis

Bacterial meningitis is an infectious process involving the dura, leptomeninges, and CSF. Although it is the most common infectious spinal disorder in children, imaging studies are usually not required, and the condition is diagnosed and treated on a clinical and physical examination basis. Infectious agents may enter the CNS through hematogenous spread, direct implantation (usually traumatic), local extension (secondary to sinusitis, mastoiditis, otitis, brain abscesses), and spread along the peripheral nervous system. Causes vary with patient age. In neonates, *Streptococcus* group B infections account for nearly 50% of cases, followed by *Escherichia coli* and *Listeria*. In young infants, *Haemophilus influenzae*

accounts for about 40% to 60% of cases, followed by *Neisseria meningitidis* and *Pneumococcus*. In older children and adults, *Pneumococcus*, *N meningitidis*, and staphylococci are the main causative agents.

The hallmark of acute-stage bacterial meningitis is arachnoiditis (ie, infiltration of the arachnoid with inflammatory cells). In this stage, a purulent exudate diffusely covers the surface of the brain and spinal cord, resulting in enhancement of the surface of the spinal cord and nerve roots on contrast-enhanced MR imaging (**Fig. 8**). Imaging studies are usually reserved for patients suspected of having complications from the disease, rather than for establishment of the diagnosis. However, neuroimaging has allowed early and precise causal diagnosis, monitoring of treatment, and identification of complications, thereby resulting in decreased morbidity and mortality. On imaging, differential diagnosis is diffuse leptomeningeal carcinomatosis (so-called neoplastic leptomeningitis). However, diffuse leptomeningeal

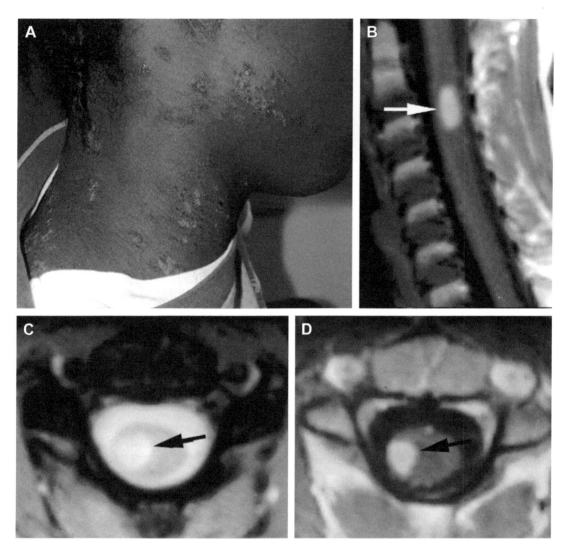

Fig. 7. Herpes zoster myelitis. (A) A patient showing shingles involving the right side of the face and neck. (B) Gd-enhanced sagittal T1-weighted image, (C) axial gradient-echo T2*-weighted image, and (D) Gd-enhanced axial T1-weighted image. There is an area of demyelination involving the right lateral spinal cord bundle at level of C3 (arrow, C), showing marked gadolinium enhancement (arrow, B, D). (Courtesy of [B–D] M. Castillo, MD, Chapel Hill, NC.)

carcinomatosis occurs only in the presence of CNS malignancy.

Acute Demyelinating Polyradiculoneuritis (Guillain-Barré Syndrome)

GBS is an acute inflammatory demyelinating disorder involving the spinal and peripheral nerves.[21,22] It is presumably caused by a prior viral disease, and such a prodromal illness, usually a respiratory illness or gastroenteritis within 2 weeks before onset, may be identified in about 65% of patients; an autoimmune mechanism directed against Schwann cells is considered to play an important role.

GBS usually occurs in children, especially boys, between 4 and 12 years of age. Clinically, it is characterized by acute onset of lower extremity weakness, progressing to paralysis and ascending to involve the upper limbs, diaphragm, and possibly cranial nerves. Sensory disturbances may be present in up to 40% of cases, and are represented by pain (perhaps the earliest clinical symptom) and paresthesia. Paralysis of the respiratory muscles is a common complication. GBS progresses rapidly, then plateaus, and resolves or improves over a period of 2 to 18 months.

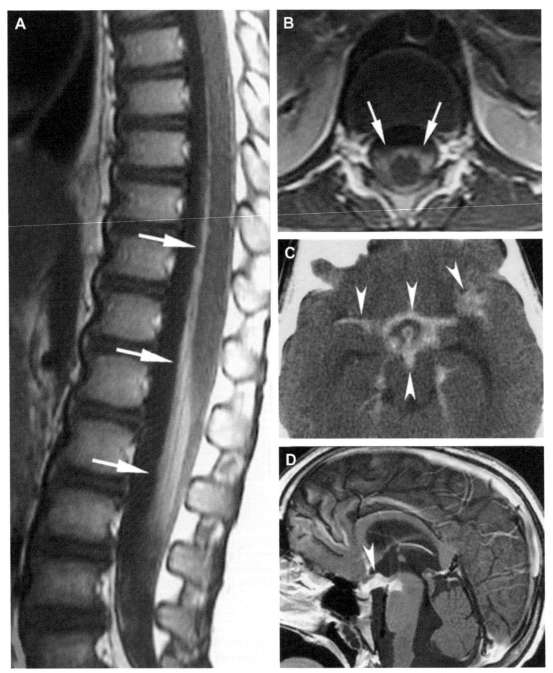

Fig. 8. Tubercular leptomeningitis. (*A*) Gd-enhanced sagittal T1-weighted image, (*B*) Gd-enhanced axial T1-weighted image, (*C*) Contrast-enhanced axial computed tomography (CT) scan, and (*D*) Gd-enhanced sagittal T1-weighted image. There is thick enhancement of the leptomeninges surrounding the spinal cord and nerve roots (*arrows, A, B*). Brain imaging also reveals thick basal leptomeningitis (*arrowheads, C, D*).

On histology, there is marked segmental demyelination and acute perivenular mononuclear cell infiltration. The nerves become thick and swollen. CSF analysis shows increase of protein levels during the initial part of the disease and a lack of inflammatory cells. If the weakness becomes progressive and lasts for more than 2 months, the patients are said to have a chronic inflammatory demyelinating polyneuropathy. This type of polyneuropathy is said to comprise about 10% of pediatric neuropathies.

Plasmapheresis is effective in adults when performed early in the course of the disease; favorable results have also been reported in children.[4] Intravenous immunoglobulins are considered to be an effective and safe treatment.[4]

MR imaging findings reflect the pathology of the disease.[23] After gadolinium administration, there is enhancement predominantly of the anterior nerve roots of the cauda equina (Fig. 9). Although the nerve roots are thickened, they do not display hyperintensity on T2-weighted images. Therefore, unenhanced studies are usually inconclusive (Fig. 10). Enhancement of posterior nerve roots may also occur, to the extent that in some cases there is global thickening and enhancement of the whole cauda equina. Posterior nerve root involvement may initially prevail, especially when pain predominates. In the very early stage of disease,

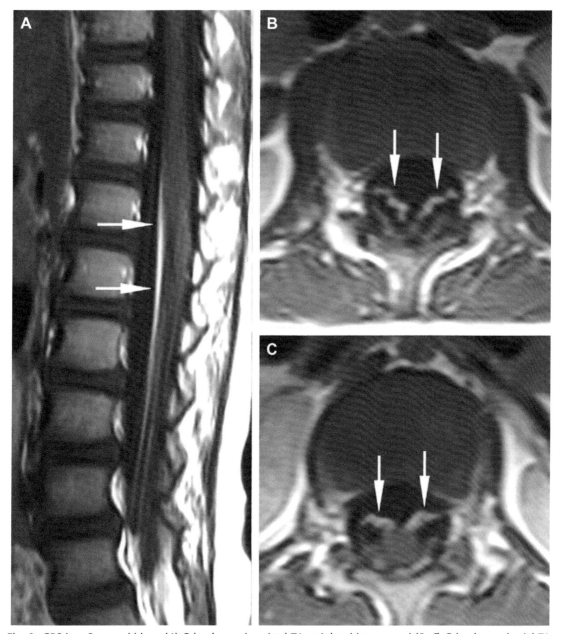

Fig. 9. GBS in a 2-year-old boy. (A) Gd-enhanced sagittal T1-weighted image, and (B, C) Gd-enhanced axial T1-weighted images. There is enhancement of the anterior nerve roots of the cauda equina (arrows, A–C). Posterior nerve roots are not involved.

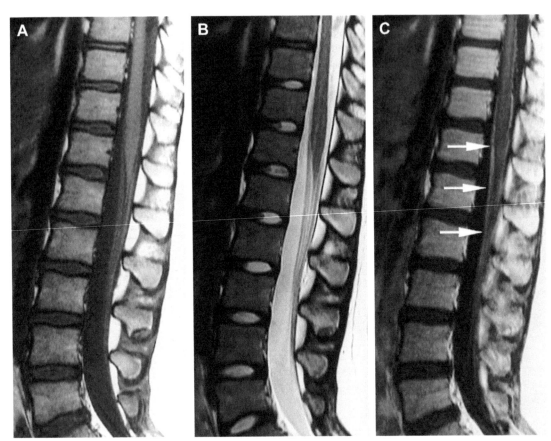

Fig. 10. GBS in a 10-year-old girl. (A) Sagittal T1-weighted image, (B) Sagittal T2-weighted image, and (C) Gd-enhanced sagittal T1-weighted image. Both unenhanced T1-weighted and T2-weighted images are unrevealing (A, B). The disorder was only disclosed by contrast-enhanced imaging (arrows, C).

enhancement may be mild, if not absent. Usually, progression to global enhancement of both anterior and posterior nerve roots occurs in a few days. On occasion, the anterior gray matter horns in the distal spinal cord also show contrast enhancement and hyperintensity on T2-weighted imaging.

Involvement of cranial nerves in the same inflammatory process is called Miller-Fisher syndrome. Affected patients present with ophthalmoplegia, ptosis, facial weakness, and ataxia. MR imaging shows enhancement of multiple cranial nerves (Fig. 11). Differential diagnosis is with neuroborreliosis (Lyme disease).

DISORDERS PREDOMINANTLY AFFECTING THE VERTEBRA, DISCS, AND EPIDURAL SPACE
Bacterial Discitis and Osteomyelitis

It is generally assumed that in children the disc is hypervascular and that infection begins there.

There is now evidence that spine infection in children generally begins in the vertebral body adjacent to the end plate in the form of microabscesses.[24] Because there are many perforating vascular channels extending into the end plate and into the disc, the infection rapidly extends into these two structures. Once the disc is involved, the infection extends again superiorly and inferiorly to affect the adjacent vertebral bodies.

Bacteriologic data are difficult to compile, because most bacterial discitis and osteomyelitis are treated on an empirical basis based on imaging study abnormalities. In addition, the incidence of discitis versus osteomyelitis is rapidly changing because of early diagnosis done using MR imaging. Despite this, staphylococci and diplococcus pneumonia account for most cases of discitis. In children with sickle cell disease, there is an increased incidence of salmonella discitis and

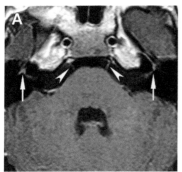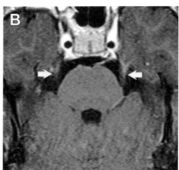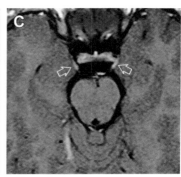

Fig. 11. Miller-Fisher syndrome in a 7-year-old boy. (A–C) Gd-enhanced axial T1-weighted images. There is symmetric enhancement of the facial nerves (*arrows, A*), abducens nerves (*arrowheads, A*), trigeminal nerves (*thick arrows, B*), and oculomotor nerves (*open arrows, C*). This patient also had diffuse enhancement of the caudal nerve roots (not shown).

osteomyelitis. In the past, osteomyelitis was more common, whereas nowadays discitis is more frequently diagnosed. Regardless of these factors, staphylococci and streptococci are the most common organisms involved.

Discitis is more commonly diagnosed between 1 and 5 years of age. Although the clinical diagnosis is straightforward, many patients present with nonspecific findings such as failure or refusal to walk, abdominal pain, chronic back pain, irritability, fever, and local tenderness. The onset of discitis may be gradual and subtle progressing over the course of 2 to 4 weeks.

MR imaging is the best method to evaluate children suspected of having spinal discitis/osteomyelitis.[25] In children, the L3-4 and L4-5 interspaces are predominantly affected. In the very early stages, imaging studies are consistent with discitis, showing a reduction in the height of the intervertebral disc associated with swelling of the annulus, which appears hyperintense in T2-weighted images. Enhancement after gadolinium administration is evident. Signal changes of the vertebral plates and subchondral regions are initially subtle. As the disease progresses, the end plates may be irregular and blurred. With advancing disease, the end plates and vertebrae become bright on T2-weighted sequences (Fig. 12). All of these abnormalities may show gadolinium enhancement. Later, infection may spread into other vertebral bodies via the venous plexus. In this situation, the adjacent vertebrae show abnormal signal intensity in the region of the canal for the basivertebral vein.

The MR imaging findings lag behind clinical improvement because of adequate antibiotic treatment. When following these patients with MR imaging, the most important feature that predicts recovery is absence of progression. The abnormalities may remain stable or improve slightly with the passing of time. Progression of disease indicates a failure of medical treatment.

Tubercular Spondylodiscitis

Spinal tuberculosis is common in children, particularly in Third World countries, although there has recently been a recrudescence of the disease in Western countries. As opposed to the adult form of the disease, childhood tuberculosis is generally more extensive and results in large abscess formation. Unlike adult tuberculosis, children seldom develop paraplegia.[26] The disease is caused by *Mycobacterium tuberculosis*. Although infection in the chest and/or genitourinary tract precedes spinal involvement in most patients, spinal involvement may be the initial manifestation of disease in children.

According to the location of the infection, 3 patterns have been described: anterior, paradiscal, and central.

In the anterior type (Fig. 13), infection begins in the anterior (and generally also inferior) vertebral body, and extends under the anterior longitudinal ligament to involve other vertebrae. The disc space can be spared, with narrowing but substantial lack of enhancement. Huge prevertebral or paravertebral abscesses originate from the vertebrae. In the paradiscal type (Fig. 14), infection begins in the lateral sides of the disc and results in narrowing of the disc space. Paradiscal disease is the least common form in children. In this case, abscesses originate directly from the disk space. In the central type (Fig. 15), infection begins in the middle of the vertebral body, may produce a vertebra plana, and eventually results in acute angle kyphosis. Central infection has a tendency to propagate posteriorly to the spinal canal, causing thecal sac compression.

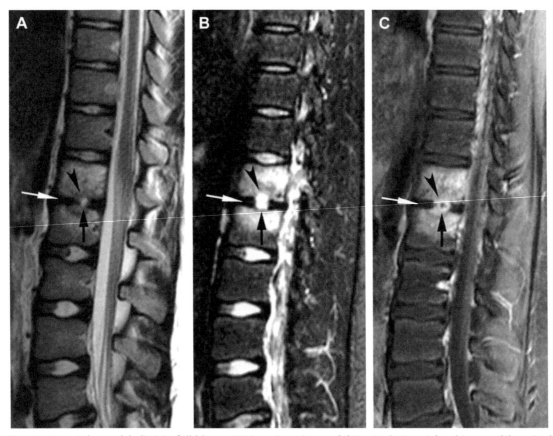

Fig. 12. Bacterial spondylodiscitis: full-blown MR imaging picture. (*A*) Sagittal T2-weighted image, (*B*) sagittal short tau inversion recovery (STIR) image, and (*C*) Gd-enhanced, fat-suppressed sagittal T1-weighted image. The disc space is narrowed (*white arrow, A–C*). The central portion of the disc is markedly hyperintense (*black arrow, A, B*) and enhances strongly (*black arrow, C*). Note the blurring of the vertebral endplates (*arrowheads, A–C*). There is marked hyperintensity and enhancement of the adjacent vertebral bodies. (*Courtesy of* M. Thurnher, MD, Vienna, Austria.)

The most frequent site for childhood spinal tuberculosis is the thoracolumbar junction.[27] Pain and signs of chronic infection are the most typical clinical manifestations. In one series, 76% of children affected were younger than 5 years of age, nearly 50% of children had neurologic deficits on hospital admission, 50% of patients recovered within 6 months of appropriate therapy, and paraspinal abscesses were found in 62% of patients. Diagnosis is difficult and may be confirmed only by positive histology and/or culture. Often, the diagnosis is based on clinical manifestations, radiographic findings, and response to antibiotics. Tuberculosis in the lumbosacral region is uncommon, and other causes, such as brucellosis, should be considered when this area is primarily involved.[28] Craniocervical involvement may also be seen in children, and is accompanied by significant abscess formation. Cervical involvement is almost always accompanied by neighboring nodal disease.[29]

Differential diagnosis is usually posed with spinal extradural tumors showing large effusive components, such as Ewing or undifferentiated sarcomas. A useful differential sign is the condition of the disk space, which is consistently involved by infectious processes and spared by tumor.

Epidural Abscess

An epidural abscess is a collection of pus between the bone and the dura mater.[24] In children they are more common in girls than in boys. Epidural abscesses are commonly secondary to pyogenic or tubercular discitis and osteomyelitis.[29] In the absence of discal and vertebral involvement, the infection usually is from hematogenous spread of

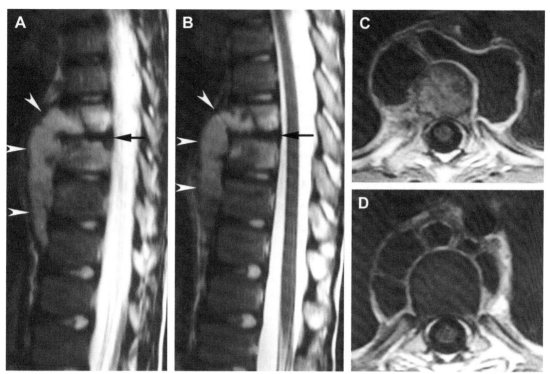

Fig. 13. Tubercular spondylodiscitis, anterior type, in an 11-year-old boy. (*A, B*) Sagittal T2-weighted images, and (*C, D*) Gd-enhanced axial T1-weighted images. There is a narrowed, hypointense disk space in the thoracic spine (*thin arrow, A, B*). Infection starts in the anterior portion of upper vertebra and generates a huge preparaverte-bral abscess (*arrowheads, A, B*; see also *C–D*). Infection propagates to the lower vertebral body, which is T2 hyperintense, as is the upper vertebral body (*A, B*).

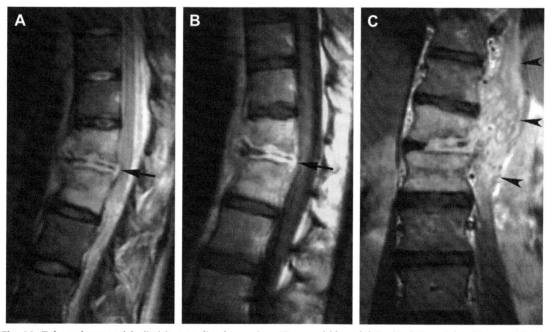

Fig. 14. Tubercular spondylodiscitis, paradiscal type, in a 13-year-old boy. (*A*) Sagittal T2-weighted image, (*B*) Gd-enhanced sagittal T1-weighted image, and (*C*) Gd-enhanced coronal T1-weighted image. There is narrowing of the disc space which appears hyperintense on T2-weighted images (*arrow, A*) and enhances markedly (*arrow, B*). Note the huge left paraspinal abscess originating from the disc space and propagating below the pillars of the diaphragm (*arrowheads, C*).

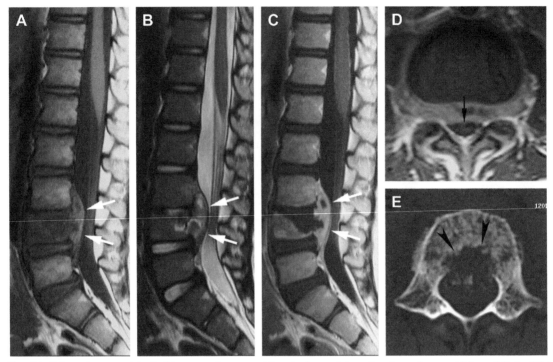

Fig. 15. Tubercular spondylodiscitis, central type, with spinal canal invasion in a 8-year-old boy. (A) Sagittal T1-weighted image, (B) sagittal T1-weighted image; (C) Gd-enhanced sagittal T1-weighted image; (D) Gd-enhanced axial T1-weighted image; and (E) axial CT scan, bone window. In this case, infection started in the central portion of the L4 vertebral body (arrowheads, E), disrupted the posterior vertebral wall, and propagated into the spinal canal below the posterior longitudinal ligament (arrows, A–C). The thecal sac is markedly compressed (arrow, D). The L3-4 disc space is irregular and probably already involved, albeit without frank, diffuse enhancement.

primary foci in the urinary tract, skin, lungs, and teeth. The most common clinical signs are pain, fever, and rapidly progressing neurologic symptoms. In children, neurologic signs may be absent or may be masked by prior administration of antibiotics.

Early on, MR imaging may detect a prominent epidural space showing intermediate signal intensity in both T1-weighted and T2-weighted images. The abnormality enhances homogeneously after gadolinium administration, and is most often a phlegmon (Fig. 16). Surgery is not indicated in these patients, because they improve considerably after appropriate antibiotic therapy. In cases of frank abscess formation, there is a rim-enhancing abnormality in the epidural space.[30] The nonenhancing center generally corresponds with pus, and surgical drainage is indicated in nearly all patients showing this type of abnormality. Abscesses are generally 2 to 4 vertebral bodies in length. In many patients with epidural abscesses, the spinal cord shows increased T2 signal intensity above, below, and at the level of the abscess. This finding is presumed to represent cord edema secondary to compromised venous drainage, secondary to involvement of the Batson plexus. Occasionally, arterial compromise with subsequent cord ischemia also occurs. The sensitivity of MR imaging for the detection of epidural abscesses is said to be more than 90%.

Chronic Recurrent Multifocal Osteomyelitis

Chronic recurrent multifocal osteomyelitis (CRMO) is a sterile skeletal inflammation occurring primarily in childhood and adolescence, predominantly in girls. The cause is unknown; autoimmune mechanisms and genetic susceptibility have been implicated.

The disease has a long, fluctuating course with exacerbations and remissions. Pain, rigidity, and malaise are the most common symptoms. Patients respond to nonsteroidal antiinflammatory drugs, whereas antibiotics are ineffective. The diagnosis is often one of exclusion in a patient with multiple localized skeletal lesions. The long-term prognosis

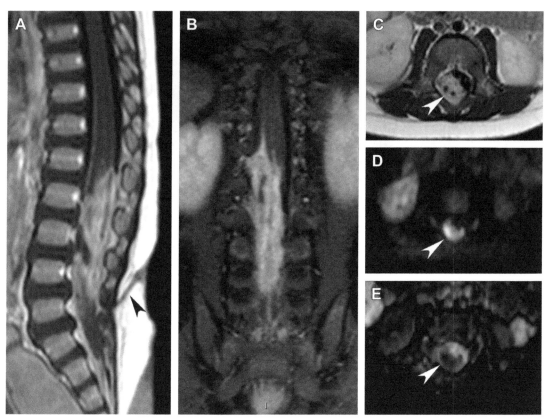

Fig. 16. Epidural phlegmon and abscess a 9-month-old girl with an infected dermal sinus. (*A*) Gd-enhanced sagittal T1-weighted image, (*B*) Gd-enhanced fat-suppressed coronal T1-weighted image, (*C*) Gd-enhanced axial T1-weighted image, (*D*) axial diffusion-weighted image, and (*E*) corresponding apparent diffusion coefficient map. In this patient with a dermal sinus (*arrowhead, A*), there is a large enhancing collection in the lumbar spinal canal (*A, B*). On axial planes, the epidural location is clearly visible (*arrowhead, C*). Note the restricted diffusion (*arrowhead, D, E*) consistent with an epidural abscess, which was confirmed at surgery.

is good.[31] Most affected children have involvement of at least 1 long bone during their illness, most frequently the femur, tibia, or pelvic bones. The spine is involved in one-third of cases at some time during concurrent illness. The vertebral involvement is often multifocal, and may occur simultaneously with involvement of other bones. The thoracic spine is involved most commonly. Vertebral collapse is not mandatory but, when present, it may progress to kyphosis and vertebra plana.

Conventional radiographs are not sensitive in the absence of clear-cut vertebral collapse, and give normal results in about 50% of cases. On computed tomography, the involved vertebrae show a mottled lytic-sclerotic appearance; on sagittal and coronal reformats, the endplates of the involved vertebrae are typically notched, giving

an impression of a wedgelike deformation. MR imaging (**Fig. 17**) shows osseous edema of the involved vertebrae, which is exquisitely depicted by short tau inversion recovery (STIR) images, and also efficiently shows endplate collapse whenever present. Spine imaging is often part of a whole-body STIR examination, which also efficiently depicts involvement in other bones.[31] The intervertebral disks are typically spared. On postcontrast T1-weighted images, enhancement of the involved vertebrae occurs, reflecting the inflammatory involvement; the use of fat-suppressed techniques is required for adequate sensitivity. Under typical conditions, the value of imaging studies is sufficient to establish a diagnosis, and vertebral biopsy is usually not necessary[32]; when performed, it shows aspecific sterile inflammation.

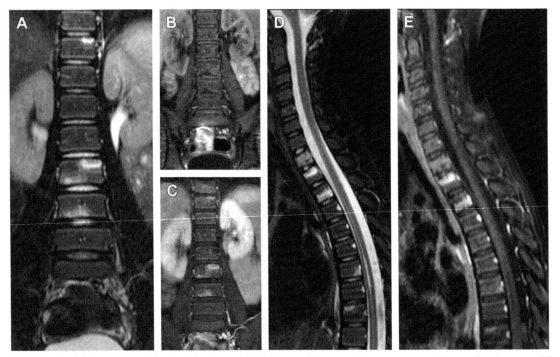

Fig. 17. CRMO in a 12-year-old girl. (*A*) Coronal STIR image, (*B*) coronal fat-suppressed T1-weighted image, (*C*) Gd-enhanced coronal fat-suppressed T1-weighted image, (*D*) sagittal STIR image, and (*E*) Gd-enhanced sagittal fat-suppressed T1-weighted image. There are multiple ill-defined areas of abnormal signal intensity involving several vertebral bodies in the whole spine. Enhancement is seen following gadolinium administration (*C*, *E*). Note that there is no vertebral collapse in this case. There is incidental hydrosyringomyelia.

REFERENCES

1. Transverse Myelitis Consortium Working Group. Proposed diagnostic criteria and nosology of acute transverse myelitis. Neurology 2002;59: 499–505.
2. Tartaglino LM, Croul SE, Flanders AE, et al. Idiopathic acute transverse myelitis: MR imaging features. Radiology 1996;201:661–9.
3. Choi KH, Lee KS, Chung SO, et al. Idiopathic transverse myelitis: MR characteristics. AJNR Am J Neuroradiol 1996;17:1151–60.
4. Smith SA, Ouvrier R. Peripheral neuropathies in children. In: Swaiman KF, Ahswal S, editors. Pediatric neurology: principles and practice. 3rd edition. St Louis (MO): Mosby; 1999. p. 1178–201.
5. Barkovich AJ. Pediatric neuroimaging. 3rd edition. Philadelphia: Lippincott Williams & Wilkins; 2000. p. 102–6.
6. Gallucci M, Caulo M, Cerone G, et al. Acquired inflammatory white matter diseases. Childs Nerv Syst 2001;17:202–10.
7. Rossi A. Imaging of acute disseminated encephalomyelitis. Neuroimaging Clin North Am 2008;18: 149–61.
8. Kaye EM. Disorders primarily affecting white matter. In: Swaiman KF, Ahswal S, editors. Pediatric neurology: principles and practice. 3rd edition. St Louis (MO): Mosby; 1999. p. 849–52.
9. Osborn AG. Diagnostic neuroradiology. St Louis (MO): Mosby; 1994.
10. Tartaglino LM, Friedman DP, Flanders AE, et al. Multiple sclerosis in the spinal cord: MR appearance and correlation with clinical parameters. Radiology 1995;195:725–32.
11. Glasier CM, Robbins MB, Davis PC, et al. Clinical, neurodiagnostic and MR findings in children with spinal and brain stem multiple sclerosis. AJNR Am J Neuroradiol 1995;16:87–95.
12. Krupp LB, Banwell B, Tenembaum S, International Pediatric MS Study Group. Consensus definitions proposed for pediatric multiple sclerosis and related disorders. Neurology 2007;68:S7–12.
13. Wingerchuk DM, Lennon VA, Lucchinetti CF, et al. The spectrum of neuromyelitis optica. Lancet Neurol 2007;6:805–15.
14. Lotze TE, Northrop JL, Hutton GJ, et al. Spectrum of pediatric neuromyelitis optica. Pediatrics 2008;122: e1039–47.

15. Trebst C, Jarius S, Berthele A, et al, Neuromyelitis Optica Study Group (NEMOS). Update on the diagnosis and treatment of neuromyelitis optica: recommendations of the Neuromyelitis Optica Study Group (NEMOS). J Neurol 2014;261:1–16.

16. DeLara F, Tartaglino L, Friedman D. Spinal cord multiple sclerosis and Devic neuromyelitis optica in children. AJNR Am J Neuroradiol 1995;16: 1557–8.

17. Murphy KJ, Brunberg JA, Quint DJ, et al. Spinal cord infection: myelitis and abscess formation. AJNR Am J Neuroradiol 1998;19:341–8.

18. Dev R, Husain M, Gupta A, et al. MR of multiple intraspinal abscesses associated with congenital dermal sinus. AJNR Am J Neuroradiol 1997;18: 742–3.

19. Malzberg MS, Rogg JM, Tate CA, et al. Poliomyelitis: hyperintensity of the anterior horn cells on MR images of the spinal cord. AJR Am J Roentgenol 1993;161:863–5.

20. Friedman DP. Herpes zoster myelitis: MR appearance. AJNR Am J Neuroradiol 1992;13:1404–6.

21. Sladky JT, Ashwal S. Inflammatory neuropathies in childhood. In: Swaiman KF, Ahswal S, editors. Pediatric neurology: principles and practice. 3rd edition. St Louis (MO): Mosby; 1999. p. 1202–15.

22. Thomas PK, Landon DN. Disease of the peripheral nerves. In: Graham DI, Lantos PL, editors. Greenfield's neuropathology, vol. 2, 6th edition. London: Arnold; 1997. p. 367–487.

23. Georgy BA, Chong B, Chamberlain M, et al. MR of the spine in Guillain-Barré syndrome. AJNR Am J Neuroradiol 1994;15:300–1.

24. Wenger DR, Davids JR, Ring D. Discitis and osteomyelitis. In: Weinstein SL, editor. The pediatric spine, principles and practice. New York: Raven; 1994. p. 813–36.

25. Bates DJ. Inflammatory diseases of the spine. Neuroimaging Clin North Am 1991;1:231–50.

26. Ho EK, Leong JC. Tuberculosis of the spine. In: Weinstein SL, editor. The pediatric spine, principles and practice. New York: Raven; 1994. p. 837–50.

27. Shanley DJ. Tuberculosis of the spine: imaging features. AJR Am J Roentgenol 1995;164:659–64.

28. Sharif HS, Clark DC, Aabed MY, et al. Granulomatous spinal infections: MR imaging. Radiology 1990;177:101–7.

29. Ruiz A, Post MJ, Ganz WI. Inflammatory and infectious processes of the cervical spine. Neuroimaging Clin North Am 1995;5:401–26.

30. Sandhu FS, Dillon WP. Spinal epidural abscess: evaluation with contrast-enhanced MR imaging. AJNR Am J Neuroradiol 1991;12:1087–93.

31. Falip C, Alison M, Boutry N, et al. Chronic recurrent multifocal osteomyelitis (CRMO): a longitudinal case series review. Pediatr Radiol 2013;43:355–75.

32. Fritz J, Tzaribatchev N, Claussen CD, et al. Chronic recurrent multifocal osteomyelitis: comparison of whole-body MR imaging with radiography and correlation with clinical and laboratory data. Radiology 2009;252:842–51.

Pyogenic Spinal Infections

E. Turgut Tali, MD*, A. Yusuf Oner, MD, A. Murat Koc, MD

KEYWORDS

- Pyogenic • Spinal Infection • Imaging

KEY POINTS

- With increasing immune suppression and globalization, spinal pyogenic infections are increasing in incidence.
- MR imaging is the modality of choice in the imaging work-up of pyogenic spinal infections.
- Characteristic imaging findings together with microbiological isolation of the causative agent are the main tools for appropriate diagnosis.
- Radiologists play an important role, because early diagnosis and treatment monitoring are extremely important in preventing morbidity and fatality.

INTRODUCTION

Pyogenic spinal infection is a life-threatening neurologic condition encompassing a broad range of clinical entities, including spondylitis, spondylodiskitis, septic diskitis, pyogenic facet arthropathy, epidural infection-abscess, leptomeningitis, and myelitis-spinal cord abscess.[1] As a significant cause of morbidity and mortality, it is difficult to differentiate from degenerative processes, inflammatory disorders, metabolic disorders, and neoplasms. Pyogenic spinal infections have a reported incidence of 0.2 to 2 cases per 100.000 per year.[2,3] Men seem to be affected twice as often as women, with a peak incidence in the sixth decade.[4] Globalization, improved life expectancy, comorbid factors, such as diabetes mellitus, drug abuse, overuse of antibiotics, immune suppression, malignancy, chronic diseases, spinal instrumentation, and increased awareness together with highly performing advanced imaging techniques have led to a rising incidence and frequency of diagnosis of spinal infections. Hematogenous spread, direct inoculation, and contiguous spread are the main routes of spinal infection. The infection is generally unimicrobial, with *Staphylococcus aureus* the main causative agent.[5] Characteristic imaging findings together with microbiological isolation of the causative agent are the main tools for appropriate diagnosis. Radiographs, CT, scintigraphy, positron emission tomography (PET)-CT, and MR imaging can all be used for this purpose and for confirmation and localization.[1,6,7]

SPONDYLITIS AND SPONDYLODISKITIS
Background and Pathophysiology

Pyogenic spondylitis/spondylodiskitis is a bacterial infection of the spinal column, intervertebral disks in association with paraspinal soft tissue, epidural space, and/or ligaments of the extradural spine infection-extension. The infection is usually unimicrobial. *S. aureus* accounts for approximately 60% and *Enterobacter* for 30% of cases. *Klebsiella*, *Pseudomonas*, *Serratia*, and *Salmonella* (in patients with sickle cell anemia) are other common organisms.[8] *S. aureus* is known to produce hyaluronidase, which is a proteolytic enzyme causing lysis of the disk.[9] The infection source is generally from a urinary tract, pulmonary, pelvic, but also can be from a

The authors certify that there is no conflict of interest with any financial organization regarding the material discussed in the article.

Neuroradiology Division, Department of Radiology, Gazi University School of Medicine, Besevler, Cankaya 06560, Ankara, Turkey

* Corresponding author.

E-mail address: turgut.tali@gmail.com

neuroimaging.theclinics.com

cutaneous infection, intravenous (IV) injections with contaminated needles, cellulitis, fasciitis, subcutaneous abscess, or pyomyositis. Predisposing factors include diabetes mellitus; other chronic diseases, such as renal failure and cirrhosis; immunosuppressed states; and IV drug use. Organisms reach the spine by 2 main routes:

1. Hematogenous spread
2. Nonhematogenous spread

Hematogenous spread can be arterial or venous. Arterial spread is more common, as a result of septicemia, and occurs at the end arteriolar level supplying the vertebral body.[10] In adults, the disk is avascular. Hematogenous organisms arrive in vertebrae via end arteriolar arcades of metaphyseal equivalent areas. Those areas correspond to subchondral plate adjacent to the disk, particularly in the anterior part. Through the disruption of cortical bone, organisms can extend to subligamentous paravertebral epidural spaces, disk, and contiguous vertebrae.[8,11] Secondary infection, however, may occur in degenerative disk disease. Granulation tissue, with the ingrowth of vessels, may penetrate radial tears and make direct hematogenous spread of infection of the disk in these cases.[12] In children, persisting vascular channels may allow direct inoculation of the disk; thus, children initially may present with diskitis alone. Because of stretching of the anterior longitudinal ligament from diskitis, abdominal pain can be the initial presenting symptom in children.[4]

The transvenous route is another hematogenous spreading path. The epidural venous plexus within the central canal, the Batson plexus, represents a series of valveless veins that extends the length of the spinal canal. The venous spreading to the spine is of particular importance in the urinary tract and other pelvic organ infections. Because the Batson plexus is a valveless system, increasing intra-abdominal pressure allows retrograde hematogeneous spread from the pelvis and abdominal organs to the vertebral column.

Nonhematogeneous spread consists of penetrating trauma, direct exposure related to skin breakdown or open wounds, surgical procedures, and diagnostic interventions, such as lumbar puncture, epidural block, nerve block, vertebroplasty, or catheterization. Compared with hematogeneous spread, direct inoculation has a prominent predilection for the pedicle, laminae, and spinous processes.[13]

Clinical Presentation

The diagnosis of pyogenic spondylodiskitis relies on clinical, imaging, and laboratory findings.

Spinal involvement level varies, and infections have been reported at all spinal segments.[3,14] The anatomic site of predilection is the lumbar region, with a frequency decreasing caudocranially over the spinal column.[15] Usually there is a delay of 2 to 12 weeks in diagnosis, which can lead to bony destruction, kyphosis, and subsequent neurologic complications.[3,16] Depending on the location and extent of the infectious process, symptoms and neurologic deficits may vary. Persistent back pain aggravated by motion, malaise, fever, anorexia, tenderness, and rigidity may be the presenting symptom. A more insidious onset with only back pain and discomfort is also possible. On physical examination, signs of nerve root compression with radiculopathy, meningeal irritation, lower extremity weakness, or paraplegia can be present with epidural involvement. Difficulty in swallowing is also another symptom in patients with cervical pyogenic spondylitis and retropharyngeal abscess. If untreated, there is an overall mortality ranging between 18% and 31%.[17]

Laboratory Tests

An initial work-up consisting of white blood cell (WBC) count, erythrocyte sedimentation rate (ESR), C-reactive protein (CRP) level, Gram stain, and blood culture should be performed for each patient suspected of pyogenic spondylitis. Together with blood culture and Gram staining, elevated ESR and CRP levels are reported as good markers of infection. ESR is found elevated in 70% to 100% of infections, and average ESR in patients with pyogenic spondylitis ranges between 43 and 87 mm per hour.[18,19] Elevated ESR, however, is not specific for infection and its use in following disease progression should be cautioned because it normalizes in an irregular and slow fashion, even after successful treatment.[3] WBC count is elevated in only 13% to 60% of cases in a moderate fashion. Although not crucial in the diagnosis, WBC count can provide general guidance in evaluating treatment response.[20] Knowing that pyogenic spondylodiskitis has a variable source of infection, blood culture, urine culture, and chest radiograph should be obtained to look for a subclinical remote infection or septicemia.

When used together with clinical findings, laboratory tests can help differentiate types of infectious spondylodiskitis. Patients with pyogenic spondylodiskitis usually present with a sharp tenderness at the site, together with spiking fevers, whereas granulomatous infection presents with a dull achy pain accompanied by a low-grade fever. Elevated ESR, CRP, and WBC counts with a shift of polymorphonuclear neutrophils to the left are present in pyogenic infections, whereas a normal to decreased WBC count together with more moderately elevated ESR and CRP is found in those with granulomatous infection.[4]

Using open or image-guided biopsy in the absence of positive blood culture for definitive microscopic or bacteriologic examination is somewhat controversial. It has been reported that 30% of percutaneous and 14% of open biopsies turned out to be false negative. To increase this biopsy yield, core biopsy should be preferred over fine-needle aspiration, and the biopsy location should be direct bone or the bony end plate instead of paravertebral soft tissue or disk.[4,14,21–23]

Imaging Evaluation

Radiographs have been used as the first step of imaging. Sensitivity and specificity of the plain films are low and are insensitive in the detection of early disease. Infection results in replacement of the normal bony matrix, resulting in a decreased vertebral bony density and lysis. This bone loss requires a 30% to 40% depletion of the bony matrix to be visible on plain radiographs, which may take approximately 2 weeks after acute onset of infection.[24] Thus, a negative plain film does not exclude the presence of spinal infection. Earliest x-ray sign is a loss of definition and irregularity of the antero-superior vertebral end plate occurring at 2 to 8 weeks. An initial increase, which can seldom be documented, and a subsequent decrease of disk height are the followers. End plate erosion is usually difficult to notice but is reported to be the most reliable radiographic sign.[25] Prevertebral and/or paravertebral soft tissue densities also may be seen. After 4 months, in the chronic stage, reactive changes in the form of sclerosis, new bone formation, osteophytes, kyphotic deformity, and bony ankylosis may ensue.

Although 3-phase technetium bone scans have a high sensitivity and specificity for spondylodiskitis, they can also be positive in osteoporotic fractures and neoplasm and they provide little anatomic detail. Because technetium is sensitive to bone remodeling, increased activity depicted on those scans can persist even after the spondylitis is healed and all laboratory findings return to normal.[26] Gallium scan is another useful nuclear medicine tool in the detection of spondylodiskitis. A combination of gallium with technetium enhances the specificity of the diagnosis and helps achieve a sensitivity of 94%. Compared with technetium, gallium scans, with a decreased sensitivity to bone remodeling, seem to be a better tool for treatment response follow-up, because they give a more accurate degree of the infectious activity.[4,26] 18-F Fluoro-deoxyglucose (FDG)-Positron emission tomography (dedicated PET) has demonstrated high sensitivity and specificity in detecting and identifying processes of inflammatory activity in spondylitis. The sensitivity, specificity, and diagnostic accuracy of FDG hybrid PET, gallium citrate GA 67, and bone scan were, respectively, 100%/87%/96%, 73%/61%/80%, and 91%/50%/80%.[27]

Although CT provides fine bone detail and increased sensitivity, it lacks specificity and cannot replace MR imaging in the diagnosis of early spondylitis and spondylodiskitis. The fine bone detail obtained from sagittal reformatted images may show lytic fragmentation, cortical erosion, sclerosis, disk hypodensity, reduced disk height, gas within the disk, soft tissue infiltration, paraspinal soft tissue swelling, and the degree of spinal canal involvement.[8,12,28] On the other hand, CT remains the preferred technique for image-guided biopsies.

MR imaging is accepted as the gold standard in imaging spinal infections. With a reported sensitivity of 96%, specificity of 92%, and accuracy of 94%, MR imaging performs better than any other radiological technique or combined nuclear medicine studies. The major strength of MR imaging is its usefulness in early detection of infection when other modalities are still normal, such as radiographs, or nonspecific, as in nuclear medicine studies.[3,20] For evaluating possible infection, MR imaging should cover the entire spinal axis and should include fat-suppressed T2-weighted imaging (T2WI) or short tau inversion recovery (STIR) images and fat-suppressed T1-weighted imaging (T1WI) to increase contrast enhancement conspicuity.[29] Infection typically begins in the anterolateral part of the vertebral body near the end plate and then spreads to involve the intervertebral disk and neighboring vertebral body.[30] The earliest sign of infection in adults is altered bone marrow signal, reflected as T2 hyperintensity, T1 hypointensity, and contrast enhancement, which is more pronounced along the end plates. Afterward, loss of definition of the end plate can be noticed. Findings of acute disk involvement are increased disk height and nonanatomic T2 hyperintensity. In the later stages of the diskitis, reduced disk height, loss of intranuclear cleft, and nonanatomic contrast enhancement are seen. Involvement of the normal disk may be missed due to its high signal on T2WI in cases without associated bony infection. Contrast administration is mandatory if there is a suspicion of infection (Fig. 1). Infection can progress and cause loss of cortical continuity of the adjacent end plates and progressive destruction of vertebral body together with soft tissue infiltration (Figs. 2 and 3), extending posteriorly

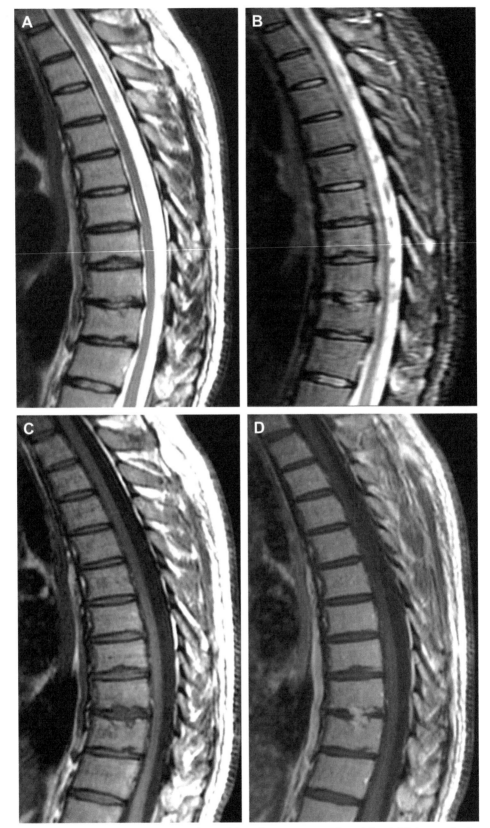

Fig. 1. Diskitis. T2-weighted (*A*), STIR (*B*), and pre- (*C*) and postcontrast T1-weighted (*D*) images in the sagittal plane show loss of the intranuclear cleft of the T9-10 disk and focal contrast enhancement consistent with pyogenic diskitis extending to the neighboring end plates.

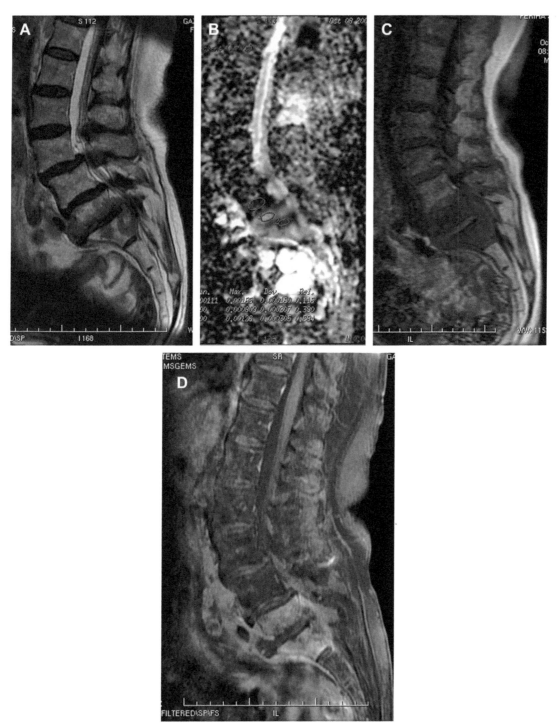

Fig. 2. Pyogenic spondylodiskitis. T2-weighted (*A*), corresponding ADC map of DWI at b = 600 mm/s (*B*), and pre- (*C*) and postcontrast T1-weighted (*D*) images in the sagittal plane show loss of the intranuclear cleft of the L5-S1 disk and loss of the hypointense band of the end plates together with erosion and contrast enhancement of the disk and neighboring vertebral bodies. A measurement from the affected disk space (region of interest 2) demonstrates decreased ADC values reflecting the pus.

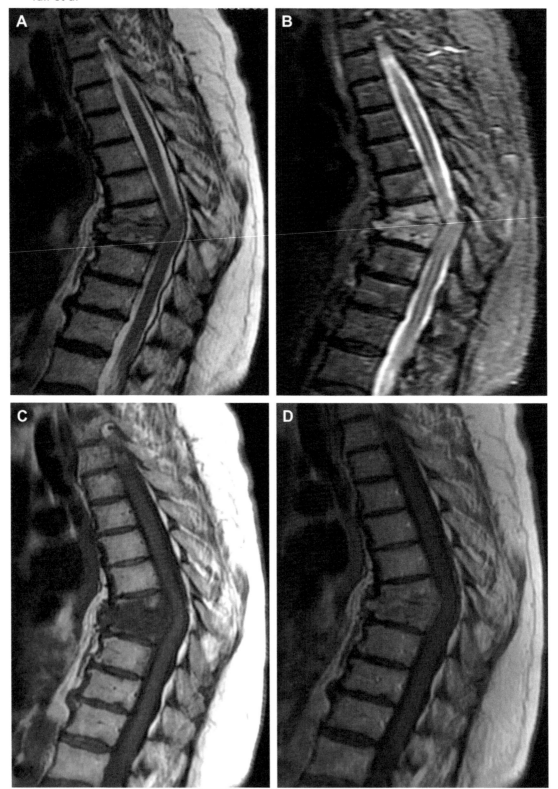

Fig. 3. Pyogenic spondylodiskitis with collapse and deformity. T2-weighted (*A*), STIR (*B*), and pre- (*C*) and post-contrast T1-weighted (*D*) images in the sagittal plane show hypointense T1, increased T2 signal and contrast enhancement within T6-7 disk space and also neighboring vertebral bodies. There is also decrease in height of the T6 and T7 vertebral bodies, together with narrowed disk space showing enhancement and causing kyphosis with mild cord compression.

into the epidural space and laterally into the paraspinal area. Articular processes and facet joints may be involved during the later stages. Reactive bone changes, new bone formation, sclerosis, kyphosis, and ankylosis are the late stage changes of the infectious process. In children, because the intervertebral disks can be directly inoculated, decreased disk height and contrast enhancement are the initial findings, followed by demineralization of adjacent vertebrae, end plate irregularities, and contiguous vertebral destruction.[8] Overall findings yielding high sensitivity in diagnosing pyogenic spondylodiskitis are vertebral bone marrow edema, disk space T2 hyperintensity, disk enhancement, and epidural/paraspinal inflammation (**Box 1**).[13,31] In addition to these findings, pyogenic spondylodiskitis may present with atypical findings, such as lack of early bone marrow signal and end plate changes, involvement of a single or adjacent 2 vertebral bodies without the intervening disk, and discrete enhancing bony lesions mimicking metastasis.[32,33] Combining clinical and laboratory information with MR imaging findings is important in solving those equivocal cases.

Although MR imaging is accepted as the gold standard in imaging spine infection, it is not without challenges, such as in treatment response follow-up. It has been reported that MR imaging can lag behind the clinical picture with a delay of 4 to 8 weeks, even months after the initiation of antibiotherapy and disease response. Focal reinstitution of T1 signal hyperintensity in the bone marrow, reflecting bone marrow recovery with fatty infiltration, or decreased or absent contrast enhancement has been suggested as a marker of healing at MR imaging follow-up (**Box 2, Fig. 4**). Still, MR imaging is not a fully reliable technique in evaluating treatment response, especially in those patients who show clinical improvement on antibiotic treatment.[24,33] Interpretation of MR imaging findings can also be challenging in the setting of postoperative spondylitis/spondylodiskitis. It has been reported that 2 parallel thin bands of enhancement in the disk

---

Box 1
Classic imaging findings of pyogenic spondylodiskitis

Invariably reduced disk height, non-anatomic T2 hyperintense, and enhancing disk

Irregularity, destruction, and enhancement of end plates and adjacent vertebral bodies

Epidural extension; phlegmon or abscess, or reactive enhancement

Soft tissue changes around spine: inhomogeneous paraspinal inflammatory swelling, abscess

---

Box 2
Imaging findings in treatment monitoring of pyogenic spondylodiskitis

Reduction of paravertebral soft tissue

Decrease of high marrow signal on STIR

Decrease of high T2 disk signal with stable disk space

Resolution of canal compromise

Progressive resolution of contrast enhancement

Increasing or persistent enhancement despite clinical improvement does not indicate treatment failure

---

space and/or paravertebral enhancement may favor spondylodiskitis over postoperative changes. Knowing that even uncomplicated postoperative spine can demonstrate disk or end plate signal changes together with enhancement, however, MR imaging cannot be used confidently in the differentiation of infection from postsurgical changes until at least 6 months after surgery.[34,35] Pleural effusion also may be seen accompanying thoracal spondylitis. The possibility of spondylitis should be considered in the patients with pleural effusion of unknown cause. Pleural effusions may be sterile in majority of accompanying spondylodiskitis.

Differential Diagnosis

When the disk space is involved, tuberculous spondylitis can resemble pyogenic spondylodiskitis. Well-defined, larger collections; paraspinal cold abscesses with thin wall sparing the disk space; skip lesions involving multiple levels by subligamentous spread; and entire vertebral body or posterior element involvement are radiological findings that support tuberculous spondylitis.[36,37] Among several noninfective conditions that can mimic pyogenic spondylodiskitis, Modic type 1 degeneration is of clinical importance and particularly challenging. Patients with Modic type 1 active end plate change are afebrile and may suffer from localized pain. On MR imaging, Modic type 1 change is characterized by T1 hypointense, T2 hyperintense signal abnormality along the vertebral end plates adjacent to a degenerated disk. Those abnormal signal intensity areas, the disk space, and the periphery of the herniated disk may enhance after IV administration of contrast media. This enhancement is attributed to ingrowth of vessels from bone into the degenerated disk and is milder compared with that seen in pyogenic spondylodiskitis. Apart from the lack of clinical features supporting infection, the hypointense nature of the degenerative disk, preservation

Initial   4 month f/u   7 month f/u   15 month f/u

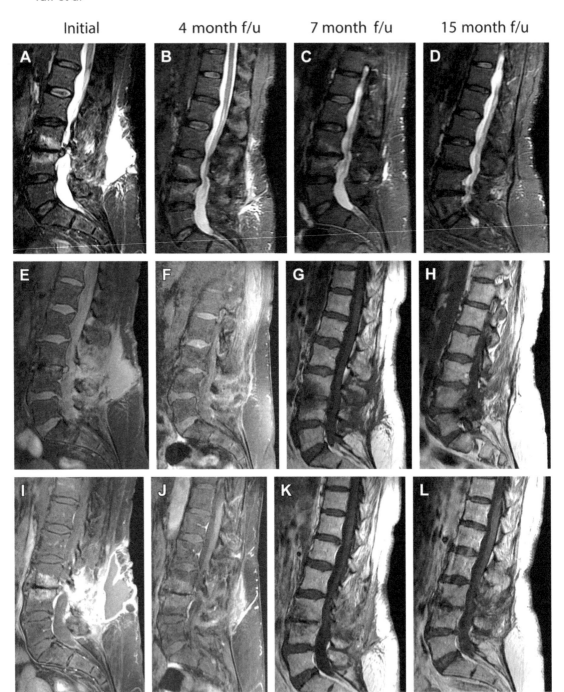

Fig. 4. Treatment monitoring of pyogenic spondylodiskitis with meningitis and paraspinal abscess. Sagittal STIR image at initial diagnosis (*A*), 4-month follow-up (*B*), 7-month follow-up (*C*), and 15-month follow-up (*D*). Respectively corresponding sagittal pre- and postcontrast T1-weighted images at initial diagnosis (*E, I*), 4-month follow-up (*F, J*), 7-month follow-up (*G, K*), and 15-month follow-up (*H, L*). Note the increased signal intensity of L3 caudal and L4 cranial end plates. Contrast enhancement of the infected areas is evident on postcontrast T1WI. Paraspinal abscess is seen with high signal intensity and peripheral enhancement on postcontrast images. Linear enhancement of the meninges consistent with meningitis is also noticed at the initial images (*I* and *J*). The follow-up images show resolution of the spondylitis, accompanying meningitis and paraspinal abscess with the successful treatment. f/u, follow-up.

of a degenerative disk space vacuum sign, preservation of vertebral end plate cortical continuity, lack of paraspinal or epidural involvement, and stability of radiological findings over time are other useful MR imaging features that can suggest Modic type 1 changes over spondylodiskitis.[8,13,29,38] Claw sign on diffusion-weighted imaging (DWI) is highly suggestive of degeneration and Modic Type 1 changes and its absence strongly suggests diskitis/osteomyelitis.[39]

Other noninfective mimics of pyogenic spondylodiskitis are dialysis arthropathy, Charcot joint, acute Schmorl node, ankylosing spondylitis, tumors, and metastasis. Dialysis arthropathy develops in patients who have been on a dialysis program for more than 3 years and resembles pyogenic spondylitis with decreased disk height and erosion of the subchondral bone. The clinical history and lack of paravertebral soft tissue infiltration are helpful in differentiation. Central and peripheral end plate erosion, thickening of the longitudinal ligament and 3-column fractures and resultant pseudoarthrosis may be seen in ankylosing spondylitis, another pyogenic spondylodiskitis mimicker. Preservation of disk space at initial stage, detection of fracture lines in the posterior elements, syndesmophytes, ligament calcification, and apophyseal joint fusions are the differential features in the later stages. Charcot arthropathy or neuropathic arthropathy of the spine is a destructive entity that may simulate spine infection. With this entity, vertebral body shows increased T2 signal and enhancement not only limited to the end plate neighboring but also encompassing its entire area, together with peripheral disk enhancement. Presence of vacuum phenomenon, involvement of facet joints, joints dislocation, spondylolisthesis, and accompanying extensive bony debris are other distinguishing features.[40,41] Acute Schmorl nodes showing enhancement with accompanying bony signal change can resemble pyogenic spondylitis. The concentric ring-type edema and involvement of the end plate adjacent to the herniated node only, with lacking diffuse disk signal abnormality, help to make the differential diagnosis.[32] Focal or diffuse signal intensity abnormality in bone marrow, hyperintense signal indicative of paravertebral soft tissue swelling, end plate irregularities, disk space narrowing, increased disk signal intensity on T2WI, and disk enhancement on postcontrast T1WI may be seen in SAPHO syndrome. Absence of the abscess or of epidural involvement and the presence of anterior vertebral corner erosion are characteristic and differentiating findings of SAPHO syndrome.[42] Diminished protective sensation of neuropathic arthropathy may cause a destructive process that occurs in response to repeated trauma. Patients with diabetes mellitus, syringomyelia, or syphilis and/or those suffering from another neuropathic disorder are prone to neuropathic arthropathy, which involves thoracolumbar junction and may mimic spondylitis. Hypointensity of the disk space and surrounding marrow on T2WI, vacuum phenomenon, and facet involvement are suggestive, however, of spinal neuropathic arthropathy.[32] Tumors and metastases are other entities that less commonly pose a diagnostic challenge. Although they may show consecutive vertebral involvement or skip lesions, tumors almost never cross the disk space and the disk height usually is preserved. Tumoral soft tissue involvement is generally well defined compared with a more diffuse pattern in spondylodiskitis.[8,26]

EPIDURAL ABSCESS
Background and Clinical Presentation

Although early reports defined the incidence of spinal epidural infection (SEI) as 0.2 to 1.96 per 10,000, recent epidemiologic studies reveal an increasing prevalence, for which early diagnosis and appropriate treatment greatly alter the clinical outcome.[1,43,44] Middle-aged men are more commonly affected and S. aureus is the most frequent pathogen.[45] Direct extension from an adjacent spondylodiskitis or facet joint infection can be a route, but epidural infections are more commonly primary, related to either hematogenous spread or iatrogenic inoculation from invasive procedures (5.5%), such as epidural block.[4] They most commonly occur in the thoracic spine and more than 70% are located in the posterior epidural space. When an epidural abscess is present in the cervical spine, it is most commonly a complication of spondylodiskitis.[46] Predisposing immunosuppressive conditions, such as diabetes mellitus, chronic renal failure, IV drug abuse, and immune deficiency may be present. Epidural abscess may present with different features, such as progressive neurologic deficit, fever, tenderness, and obtundation, but severe back pain is the most common symptom. Elevated ESR and CRP are seen more frequently than leukocytosis.[47] Functional impairment seen in epidural abscess is not only related to mechanical compression of the cord or techal sac but also to vascular mechanisms, such as thrombosis or thrombophlebitis. Once the infectious process reaches the epidural space, compression or vascular impairment of epidural veins may cause spinal venous congestion with ensuing irreversible spinal cord infarction. Hence, the detection of epidural abscess requires urgent surgical intervention.[4,48,49]

Imaging Evaluation and Differential Diagnosis

MR imaging, providing a sensitivity of 91% to 100%, is the modality of choice, and, when spinal epidural abscess is clinically suspected, imaging the entire spine is recommended.[1,47] MR imaging demonstrates a T1 hypointense, T2 hyperintense soft tissue mass within the epidural space, with hypointense thickened and displaced dura on T1WI and T2WI, causing cord or thecal sac compression. Diagnosis may be difficult when signal is similar to cerebrospinal fluid (CSF) and when meningitis and epidural infection both are present. Contrast media injection is a must and helps differentiate epidural phlegmon from abscess. Phlegmon does not contain pus, shows almost uniform enhancement, and may be treated more conservatively. On the other hand, abscess has a liquid content or pus, showing rim enhancement, and requires urgent surgical intervention (**Figs. 5** and **6**).[31,50] DWI can also be used to show the expected restriction in the abscess cavity.[51,52] Depending on the infecting agents, air also may be seen rarely. After treatment, in contrast to spondylodiskitis, imaging changes seem to correlate with the clinical course. Although diagnosis of an epidural abscess is straightforward when associated with diskitis or facet joint infection, it can be a challenge in primary cases. SEI may cause damage to spinal cord, which is out of proportion to the size of inflammation. Spinal cord damage may be due to many factors, including arterial compression, focal ischemia-infarction, edema, and venous infarction by venous thrombosis-thrombophlebitis, and also direct effects of exotoxins of the causitive agents. In these circumstances, differential consideration should include malignancy and hematoma. Apart from clinical history, the more central location of tumors, which most commonly involves the midline septum of the ventral epidural space, can help in making the correct diagnosis from an abscess.[13,53]

SUBDURAL ABSCESS

Primary subdural abscess is extremely rare and generally a secondary condition located in the lumbar region.[13] S. aureus is the most common causative pathogen. Population at risk, predisposing factors, and clinical presentation are similar to epidural abscess. On MR imaging, subdural abscess is seen as a crescent-shaped, irregular thick-walled collection showing enhancement, which may compress the nerve roots and spinal cord.[4] Subdural abscess can be easily differentiated from epidural abscess by its deeper location and the preservation of the normal thecal sac configuration. Treatment is generally surgical drainage followed by antibiotherapy.[54,55]

FACET JOINT INFECTION

Facet joint infection, once thought an uncommon condition, is increasingly recognized. Because the vascular supply of the facet joints differs from that of vertebral bodies, nonhematogenous involvement is more common than hematogenous spread, with S. aureus the main infectious agent. Besides cutaneous, respiratory, and urinary infections, minimally invasive therapeutic procedures can be the source. Population at risk, predisposing factors, and clinical presentation are similar to spondylodiskitis. The back pain is, however, typically unilateral and more acute and severe than that of pyogenic spondylodiskitis.[56,57] Bilaterality suggests transmission of the infection through the retroligamentous space of Okada.[13,58] CT, as with radiographs, is of limited utility, particularly early in the disease course, but may demonstrate erosive changes, loss of density of ligamentum flavum, and obliteration of fat planes.[59] MR imaging, including fat-suppressed images together with IV contrast injection, is the modality of choice. Swelling of the pus fluid–filled, peripherally enhancing capsule and accompanying soft tissue edema with high signal on T2WI and bony erosive changes are readily depicted on MR imaging (**Fig. 7**). Antibiotherapy is the mainstay of treatment, with surgery reserved only for cases complicated with epidural abscess or medical treatment failure.

LEPTOMENINGITIS

Pyogenic leptomeningitis is the most common bacterial infection of the spinal axis, with differing causative agents according to age: group B streptococcus, gram-negative bacilli, and Listeria in newborns; Haemophilus influenzae, Streptococcus pneumoniae, and Neisseria meningitidis in children between ages 2 and 12; and streptococci and staphylococci in adults.[1,6] Initially, acute inflammatory exudate lodges in subarachnoid space and toxic mediators potentiate inflammatory response and cause increased permeability of vessels. Fever, chills, headache, altered level of consciousness, neck stiffness, paraparesis, paresthesia, gait disturbance, and urinary bladder dysfunction are the clinical findings of the acute stage.

MR imaging is the modality of choice and contrast is essential. MR imaging without contrast may be entirely normal at the acute stage whereas

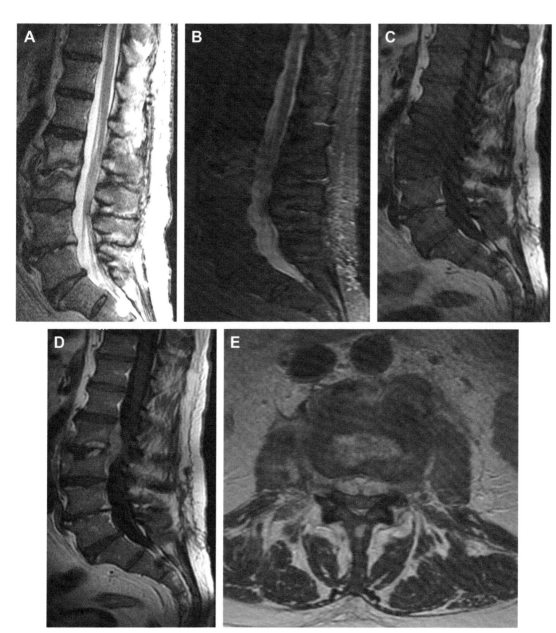

Fig. 5. Pyogenic spondylodiskitis with epidural phlegmon. T2-weighted (*A*), STIR (*B*), and pre- (*C*) postcontrast T1-weighted (*D*) images in the sagittal plane and postcontrast T1-weighted axial image (*E*) show erosion and destruction of the neighboring end plates of L2-3 disk space together with increased disk signal. Affected vertebral bodies are hypointense on T1- and hyperintense on T2WI. Enhancement is also noticed. The extension of the spondylodiskitis obliterates the anterior epidural space by homogeneously enhancing phlegmon formation, which is compressing the thecal sac.

contrast-enhanced MR imaging has findings. Pathologic contrast enhancement of the meninges and nerve root sheaths are pathognomonic for the spinal meningitis. Linear, focal-nodular, patchy contrast enhancement may be seen. The opposite is valid for the chronic stage of the spinal meningitis because unenhanced MR imaging may show findings whereas there may not be contrast enhancement. The pattern of enhancement, however, has no significant correlation with the severity of symptoms and has no specific value in differentiating infection from leptomeningeal tumoral infiltration.[60] In the advanced stages, loss of definition between cord and CSF, thickening of the meninges, obliteration of low signal area of CSF, meningeal adhesions, and obliteration of the CSF space with filled

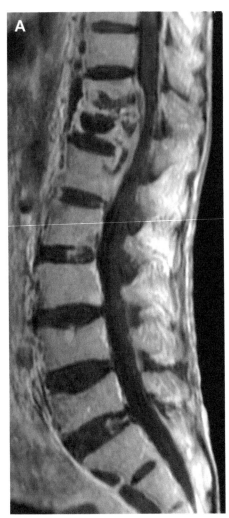
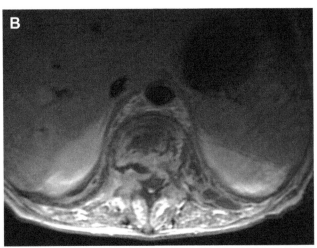

Fig. 6. Pyogenic spondylodiskitis with collapse, epidural extension, and abscess formation. Postcontrast T1WIs in the sagittal (*A*) and axial planes (*B*) show enhancing foci of spondylodiskitis at the thoracolomber junction with kyphosis due to collapsed Th11 and Th12 thoracic vertebral bodies. The infection extends to the anterior epidural space with peripherally enhancing abscess causing mild cord and thecal sac compression.

exudate and dilated vessels may cause loculations. Thickened roots and plastering and clumping of the roots also may be seen commonly. Extensive exudate with accompanying vasculitis more prominently in veins may cause cord ischemia and infarction. Vessels into and traversing exudate may be infected and cause venous congestion and edema of the spinal cord and myelitis. Spinal meningitis also may cause spinal cord and nerve root compression, spinal cord demyelination, myelomalacia, myelopathy, myelitis, and necrosis. Impaired CSF flow may cause syringomyelia or cystic changes into the spinal cord. Metastasis, sarcoidosis, intracranial hypotension, subdural hematoma, Guillain-Barré syndrome, and idiopathic

hypertrophic spinal pachymeningitis should be ruled out as the differential diagnosis.

MYELITIS AND SPINAL CORD ABSCESS

Spinal cord infection is uncommon and associated with high morbidity and mortality. Hematogenous spread, extension from brain, meninges, and adjacent spondylodiskitis are main routes of transmission. Congenital defects and dermal sinus are frequently present, particularly in pediatric patients presenting with myelitis and spinal cord abscess. Clinical presentation may be acute or chronic and can result in progressive neurologic decline. In the acute stages, which are less than

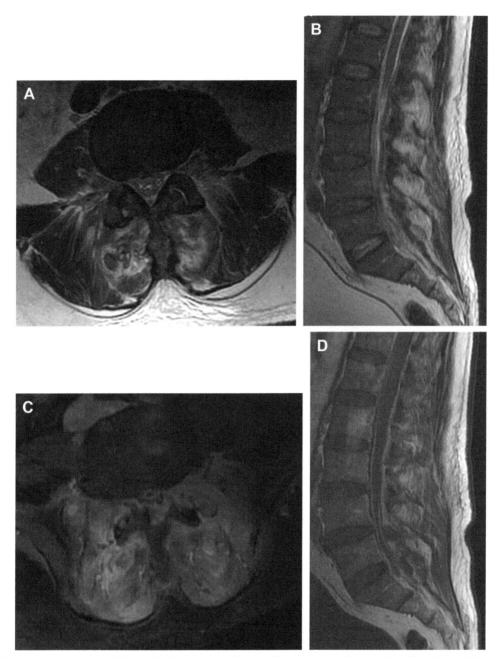

Fig. 7. Pyogenic spondylodiskitis with leptomeningitis and facet joint septic arthritis. T2-weighted (*A, B*) and postcontrast T1-weighted (*C, D*) images in the axial and sagittal planes, respectively, show thickening and contrast enhancement of the meninges, nerve root sheaths consistent with leptomeningitis. There is also pus-filled, swelled, peripherally enhancing facet joint, with subarticular bony erosive changes and soft tissue edema depicting accompanying facet joint septic arthritis.

a week, a triad of fever, pain, and neurologic deficit is the hallmark. Motor deficit, sensory disturbance, sphincter dysfunction, and meningismus may accompany with the laboratory findings of leukocytosis and elevated ESR. In the chronic stage, more than 6 weeks after the onset, fever is not seen whereas varying degrees of neurologic deterioration are common. WBC counts turn to normal with continuing elevated ESR.

MR imaging is also the gold standard for diagnosis of myelitis and spinal cord abscesses. There is hypointensity on T1WI and

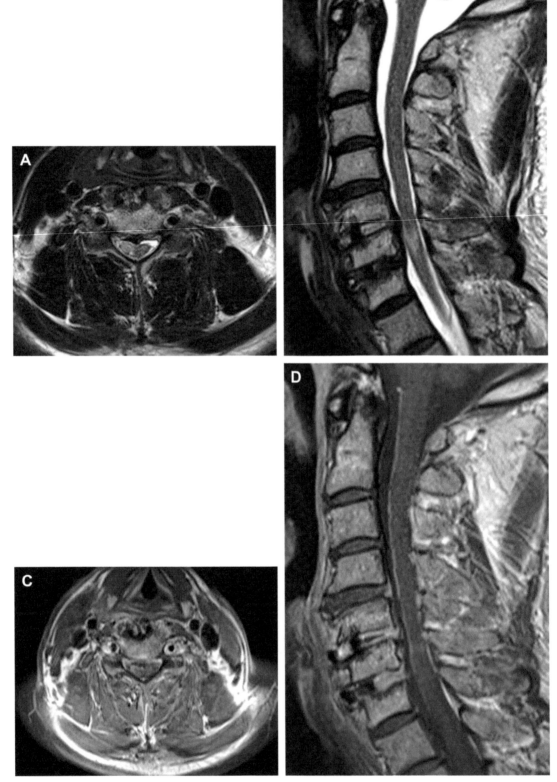

Fig. 8. Pyogenic spondylodiskitis with leptomeningitis and myelitis. T2- weighted (*A, B*) and postcontrast T1-weighted (*C, D*) images in the axial and sagittal planes, respectively, in a patient with previous history of cervical disk surgery. Nodular contrast enhancement is seen at the C5-6, C6-7 intervertebral disk spaces together with meningeal enhancement. Edema and focal swelling at the right half of the cord is also present. Contrast enhancement is noticed at the corresponding area of the cord.

hyperintensity on T2WI due to edema whereas the infected area shows slightly less hyperintensity on T2WI than edema in a nonvascular distribution. The spinal cord may show diffuse or fusiform enlargement with or without skip areas. Contrast enhancement may change from mild to marked and may be homogeneous or heterogeneous (Fig. 8). MR imaging findings of spinal cord abscess may present edema and diffuse, patchy, or ring enhancement consistent with the stage of infection, together with central diffusion restriction and low apparent diffusion coefficient (ADC) signal and values.[1,4,61]

Differential diagnosis of myelitis–spinal cord abscess consists of acute transverse myelitis, inflammatory lesions as multiple sclerosis, ischemia-infarct, syringohydromyelia, cystic lesions, primary or secondary neoplasia, and vascular malformations.

SUMMARY

In the era of immune suppression, tuberculosis, and the HIV epidemic, together with worldwide socioeconomic fluctuations giving rise to new homeless populations, spinal infections are increasing in incidence. Early diagnosis and treatment require correlation of patient history, physical examination findings, and imaging features to prevent morbidity and fatality. Radiologists play an important role in this potentially fatal condition, with contrast-enhanced MR imaging the modality of choice. This article provides an imaging overview that can help in prompt and correct diagnosis of pyogenic spinal infections.

REFERENCES

1. Tali ET, Gultekin S. Spinal infections. Eur Radiol 2005;15(3):599–607.
2. Kapeller P, Fazekas F, Krametter D, et al. Pyogenic infectious spondylitis: clinical, laboratory and MRI features. Eur Neurol 1997;38(2):94–8.
3. Cheung WY, Luk KD. Pyogenic spondylitis. Int Orthop 2012;36(2):397–404.
4. Go JL, Rothman S, Prosper A, et al. Spine infections. Neuroimaging Clin N Am 2012;22(4):755–72.
5. Yoon SH, Chung SK, Kim KJ, et al. Pyogenic vertebral osteomyelitis: identification of microorganism and laboratory markers used to predict clinical outcome. Eur Spine J 2010;19(4):575–82.
6. Baleriaux DL, Neugroschl C. Spinal and spinal cord infection. Eur Radiol 2004;14(Suppl 3):E72–83.
7. Mellado JM, Perez del Palomar L, Camins A, et al. MR imaging of spinal infection: atypical features, interpretive pitfalls and potential mimickers. Eur Radiol 2004;14(11):1980–9.
8. Tali ET. Spinal infections. Eur J Radiol 2004;50(2):120–33.
9. Jinkins JR, Bazan C 3rd, Xiong L. MR of disc protrusion engendered by infectious spondylitis. J Comput Assist Tomogr 1996;20(5):715–8.
10. Sapico FL. Microbiology and antimicrobial therapy of spinal infections. Orthop Clin North Am 1996;27(1):9–13.
11. Van Tassel P. Magnetic resonance imaging of spinal infections. Top Magn Reson Imaging 1994;6(1):69–81.
12. Stabler A, Reiser MF. Imaging of spinal infection. Radiol Clin North Am 2001;39(1):115–35.
13. Diehn FE. Imaging of spine infection. Radiol Clin North Am 2012;50(4):777–98.
14. Jaramillo-de la Torre JJ, Bohinski RJ, Kuntz CT. Vertebral osteomyelitis. Neurosurg Clin N Am 2006;17(3):339–51, vii.
15. Calderone RR, Larsen JM. Overview and classification of spinal infections. Orthop Clin North Am 1996;27(1):1–8.
16. Perronne C, Saba J, Behloul Z, et al. Pyogenic and tuberculous spondylodiskitis (vertebral osteomyelitis) in 80 adult patients. Clin Infect Dis 1994;19(4):746–50.
17. Smith AS, Blaser SI. Infectious and inflammatory processes of the spine. Radiol Clin North Am 1991;29(4):809–27.
18. Carragee EJ, Kim D, van der Vlugt T, et al. The clinical use of erythrocyte sedimentation rate in pyogenic vertebral osteomyelitis. Spine 1997;22(18):2089–93.
19. Weiser S, Rossignol M. Triage for nonspecific lower-back pain. Clin Orthop Relat Res 2006;443:147–55.
20. An HS, Seldomridge JA. Spinal infections: diagnostic tests and imaging studies. Clin Orthop Relat Res 2006;(444):27–33.
21. Visuri T, Pihlajamaki H, Eskelin M. Long-term vertebral changes attributable to postoperative lumbar discitis: a retrospective study of six cases. Clin Orthop Relat Res 2005;(433):97–105.
22. Govender S. Spinal infections. J Bone Joint Surg Br 2005;87(11):1454–8.
23. Yee DK, Samartzis D, Wong YW, et al. Infective spondylitis in Southern Chinese: a descriptive and comparative study of ninety-one cases. Spine 2010;35(6):635–41.
24. Gillams AR, Chaddha B, Carter AP. MR appearances of the temporal evolution and resolution of infectious spondylitis. AJR Am J Roentgenol 1996;166(4):903–7.
25. Mahboubi S, Morris MC. Imaging of spinal infections in children. Radiol Clin North Am 2001;39(2):215–22.
26. Tyrrell PN, Cassar-Pullicino VN, McCall IW. Spinal infection. Eur Radiol 1999;9(6):1066–77.
27. Gratz S, Dorner J, Fischer U, et al. 18F-FDG hybrid PET in patients with suspected spondylitis. Eur J Nucl Med Mol Imaging 2002;29(4):516–24.

28. Darden BV 2nd, Duncan J. Postoperative lumbar spine infection. Orthopedics 2006;29(5):425–9 [quiz: 430–1].

29. Longo M, Granata F, Ricciardi K, et al. Contrast-enhanced MR imaging with fat suppression in adult-onset septic spondylodiscitis. Eur Radiol 2003;13(3):626–37.

30. Modic MT, Feiglin DH, Piraino DW, et al. Vertebral osteomyelitis: assessment using MR. Radiology 1985;157(1):157–66.

31. Dagirmanjian A, Schils J, McHenry M, et al. MR imaging of vertebral osteomyelitis revisited. AJR Am J Roentgenol 1996;167(6):1539–43.

32. Hong SH, Choi JY, Lee JW, et al. MR imaging assessment of the spine: infection or an imitation? Radiographics 2009;29(2):599–612.

33. Hsu CY, Yu CW, Wu MZ, et al. Unusual manifestations of vertebral osteomyelitis: intraosseous lesions mimicking metastases. AJNR Am J Neuroradiol 2008;29(6):1104–10.

34. Ross JS, Zepp R, Modic MT. The postoperative lumbar spine: enhanced MR evaluation of the intervertebral disk. AJNR Am J Neuroradiol 1996;17(2):323–31.

35. Van Goethem JW, Parizel PM, van den Hauwe L, et al. The value of MRI in the diagnosis of postoperative spondylodiscitis. Neuroradiology 2000;42(8):580–5.

36. Early SD, Kay RM, Tolo VT. Childhood diskitis. J Am Acad Orthop Surg 2003;11(6):413–20.

37. Wang D. Diagnosis of tuberculous vertebral osteomyelitis (TVO) in a developed country and literature review. Spinal Cord 2005;43(9):531–42.

38. Zhang YH, Zhao CQ, Jiang LS, et al. Modic changes: a systematic review of the literature. Eur Spine J 2008;17(10):1289–99.

39. Patel KB, Poplawski MM, Pawha PS, et al. Diffusion-weighted MRI "claw sign" improves differentiation of infectious from degenerative modic type 1 signal changes of the spine. AJNR Am J Neuroradiol 2014;35(8):1647–52.

40. Wagner SC, Schweitzer ME, Morrison WB, et al. Can imaging findings help differentiate spinal neuropathic arthropathy from disk space infection? Initial experience. Radiology 2000;214(3):693–9.

41. Lacout A, Lebreton C, Mompoint D, et al. CT and MRI of spinal neuroarthropathy. AJR Am J Roentgenol 2009;193(6):W505–14.

42. Laredo JD, Vuillemin-Bodaghi V, Boutry N, et al. SAPHO syndrome: MR appearance of vertebral involvement. Radiology 2007;242(3):825–31.

43. Hlavin ML, Kaminski HJ, Ross JS, et al. Spinal epidural abscess: a ten-year perspective. Neurosurgery 1990;27(2):177–84.

44. Khan SH, Hussain MS, Griebel RW, et al. Title comparison of primary and secondary spinal epidural abscesses: a retrospective analysis of 29 cases. Surg Neurol 2003;59(1):28–33 [discussion: 33].

45. Reihsaus E, Waldbaur H, Seeling W. Spinal epidural abscess: a meta-analysis of 915 patients. Neurosurg Rev 2000;23(4):175–204 [discussion: 205].

46. James SL, Davies AM. Imaging of infectious spinal disorders in children and adults. Eur J Radiol 2006;58(1):27–40.

47. Tompkins M, Panuncialman I, Lucas P, et al. Spinal epidural abscess. J Emerg Med 2010;39(3):384–90.

48. Feldenzer JA, McKeever PE, Schaberg DR, et al. The pathogenesis of spinal epidural abscess: microangiographic studies in an experimental model. J Neurosurg 1988;69(1):110–4.

49. Darouiche RO. Spinal epidural abscess. N Engl J Med 2006;355(19):2012–20.

50. Tang HJ, Lin HJ, Liu YC, et al. Spinal epidural abscess–experience with 46 patients and evaluation of prognostic factors. J Infect 2002;45(2):76–81.

51. Moritani T, Kim J, Capizzano AA, et al. Pyogenic and non-pyogenic spinal infections: emphasis on diffusion-weighted imaging for the detection of abscesses and pus collections. Br J Radiol 2014;87(1041):20140011.

52. Eastwood JD, Vollmer RT, Provenzale JM. Diffusion-weighted imaging in a patient with vertebral and epidural abscesses. AJNR Am J Neuroradiol 2002;23(3):496–8.

53. Kim DH, Rosenblum JK, Panghaal VS, et al. Differentiating neoplastic from nonneoplastic processes in the anterior extradural space. Radiology 2011;260(3):825–30.

54. Vural M, Arslantas A, Adapinar B, et al. Spinal subdural Staphylococcus aureus abscess: case report and review of the literature. Acta Neurol Scand 2005;112(5):343–6.

55. Kulkarni AG, Chu G, Fehlings MG. Pyogenic intradural abscess: a case report. Spine 2007;32(12):E354–7.

56. Narvaez J, Nolla JM, Narvaez JA, et al. Spontaneous pyogenic facet joint infection. Semin Arthritis Rheum 2006;35(5):272–83.

57. Weingarten TN, Hooten WM, Huntoon MA. Septic facet joint arthritis after a corticosteroid facet injection. Pain Med 2006;7(1):52–6.

58. Kotsenas AL. Imaging of posterior element axial pain generators: facet joints, pedicles, spinous processes, sacroiliac joints, and transitional segments. Radiol Clin North Am 2012;50(4):705–30.

59. Babinchak TJ, Riley DK, Rotheram EB Jr. Pyogenic vertebral osteomyelitis of the posterior elements. Clin Infect Dis 1997;25(2):221–4.

60. Rothman SL. The diagnosis of infections of the spine by modern imaging techniques. Orthop Clin North Am 1996;27(1):15–31.

61. Al Barbarawi M, Khriesat W, Qudsieh S, et al. Management of intramedullary spinal cord abscess: experience with four cases, pathophysiology and outcomes. Eur Spine J 2009;18(5):710–7.

Pediatric and Adult Spinal Tuberculosis
Imaging and Pathophysiology

Tracy Kilborn, MBChB, FRCR (UK)[a],*,
Pieter Janse van Rensburg, MBChB, FRCR (UK), MMed (RadDiag), FRCPC[b],
Sally Candy, MBChB, FcRad (Diag) SA[c]

KEYWORDS

• Spinal infection • Tuberculosis • MR imaging

KEY POINTS

• The spine is involved in up to 50% of skeletal TB cases, often presenting with advanced disease as a result of the indolent nature of the infection and low index of suspicion of the diagnosis of TB in non–TB endemic areas.
• Nonosseous TB may involve the cord, cauda equine, and/or the meninges.
• MR imaging is the imaging modality of choice in the evaluation of spinal TB and should include the whole spine, to assess for multilevel noncontiguous spinal disease.
• Including the chest and abdomen in the MR imaging aids in the diagnosis by identifying extraspinal sites of TB.

HISTORICAL PERSPECTIVE

In 1782, the English surgeon Sir Percivall Pott described the clinical presentation, examination, and pathologic findings of tuberculous spondylitis (TBS). A century later, the German physician and microbiologist Robert Koch would isolate the causative organism and receive the Nobel Prize in 1905.

PATHOGENESIS

Vertebral infection results from dissemination of the tuberculous bacilli from a distant active source or as a result of latent reactivation. Tuberculous involvement of the vertebral body may be paradiscal, anterior subperiosteal, central, or appendiceal.[1] Emphasis has been placed on the normal vascular anatomy of the spine to explain differences in the patterns of infection in children and adults and pyogenic spondylitis versus TBS.

The arterial supply of the vertebral column arises from segmental branches of the vertebral, subclavian, intercostal, and lumbar arteries. Intraosseous arteries arise from two sets of vessels, one anteriorly on the vertebral surface and the other within the spinal canal. Zoned vascular territories have been proposed: the central core of the vertebral body extending from disk to disk supplied by the equatorial arteries, an annular region near the end plate by the metaphyseal arteries, and a surrounding collar from disk to disk supplied by the penetrating arteries.[2,3]

During the second trimester the intervertebral regions of the spine are avascular. Later in fetal life there is centripetal vascular growth from the periphery and centrifugal vessel growth from the

No disclosures.
[a] Department of Pediatric Radiology, Red Cross War Memorial Children's Hospital, University of Cape Town, Klipfontein Road, Rondebosch, Cape Town 7700, South Africa; [b] Department of Medical Imaging, Regina General Hospital, College of Medicine, University of Saskatchewan, 1440-14th Avenue, Regina SK S4P 0W5, Canada; [c] Department of Radiology, Groote Schuur Hospital, University of Cape Town, Main Road, Observatory, Cape Town 7925, South Africa
* Corresponding author.
E-mail address: tracykilborn@gmail.com

ossification centers.[4] This active vascularization results in an extensive intraosseous anastomotic network in the infantile vertebral body and annulus fibrosis. The nucleus pulposis in contradistinction is never vascular. Vascularity diminishes and disappears entirely by the third decade of life resulting in intraosseous end-arteries.[5] Although these differences may be important determinants in the pathogenesis of pyogenic spine infection, their importance in TBS is less clear. The valveless craniospinal venous plexus of Batson has received recent attention as a potential route of disease and tumor spread and has been implicated in the development of noncontiguous TBS.[6–9] The central vertebral body pattern of tuberculous infection could be attributable either to the centrally located basivertebral veins or the equatorial arteries.

PATHOLOGY

Up to one-half of all musculoskeletal tuberculosis (TB) affects the spine, most commonly in the thoracic and upper lumbar levels.[10] Once the tuberculous bacilli reach the vertebral body or end plate, either hematogenously, via the lymphatics, or directly, in the absence of adequate cell-mediated immunity, active bone destruction (spondylitis) may result. Alternatively there may be partial containment with latent granuloma formation and subsequent reactivation.

The hallmark of TB is the presence of granulomatous inflammation with caseous necrosis. Phagocytosis of the organisms by macrophages results initially in granuloma formation. Central caseation and granuloma breakdown are responsible for release of bacilli into the extracellular space. Once the disease process is no longer confined, extracellular multiplication of bacilli and caseous liquefaction result in destructive spread into the neighboring tissues.[11,12]

Bone destruction and adjacent tissue necrosis form what has become known as a "pseudo" or "cold" abscess (as distinct from the true polymorph dominant abscess cavity of pyogenic infection) in a high proportion of adult and pediatric patients.[2,8,13] Spread to the extraosseous tissues is typically subjacent to the anterior and posterior longitudinal ligaments, paravertebral soft tissues, intervertebral disk, or spinal canal. Paravertebral masses may become very large and displace abdominal organs causing compressive changes in adjacent vertebral bodies. Epidural soft tissue masses are present in 60% to 93% with associated displacement of the thecal sac and compression of the cord or cauda equina.[6,13] Fistulization to distant sites is common.[6]

Posterior vertebral element involvement, especially isolated disease, is less common. Pedicle involvement as a late and secondary occurrence has been demonstrated in 68% in adults[14] and, in our experience, 85% of children. The average number of contiguous bodies affected (two to three) and the occurrence of noncontiguous disease (<20%) are similar in children and adults and do not seem to be influenced by immune compromise.[11,15] Sparing of the intervertebral disk in TB was thought to be a classic feature and one that distinguishes TBS from pyogenic spondylitis. More recently with the availability of MR imaging it is clear that disk destruction is common at presentation in TBS,[15–18] although it remains true that subligamentous extension between adjacent bodies is the primary mode of spread. Local bony destruction and subligamentous decompression may be so extensive that one or more vertebral bodies and their adjacent disks are subsumed in the abscess giving the false impression of disk sparing.

The kyphotic curvature of the spine (gibbus) described by Pott is explained by anterior vertebral body collapse. The exact reason for this is conjectural. Kyphosis may be associated with a combination of epidural pseudoabscess, bony sequestrate, retropulsed sequestered disk, vertebral subluxation/dislocation, and concertina collapse. Less commonly there may be associated penetration of the dura with meningovascular cord compromise.[11,19] Neurologic deficit tends to occur late in TBS because of the rather slow increase in pressure on the neural axis.[20] Paraplegia may occur without significant kyphosis when there is mechanical instability or vascular compromise.[20,21]

CLINICAL PRESENTATION

In a large study of 694 adult patients the commonest presenting complaint was paraplegia and/or spinal deformity (70%). Back pain and fever were less frequent (20%).[20] In children the symptoms are commonly nonspecific including torticollis, refusal to weight bear, limp, pain, and palpable mass. It should be remembered that back pain in a child is a red flag necessitating MR imaging. The diagnosis of TB can be suggested on imaging but treatment requires identification of the tuberculous bacillus, and isolation of drug sensitivities (Box 1).

IMAGING FINDINGS
Radiographs of the Spine

Despite being the mainstay of diagnosis, particularly in resource-limited settings, radiography has disadvantages. More than 50% of the

Box 1
Making the diagnosis of TB

- Mantoux tuberculin skin test (in children and unexposed adults).
- Ziehl-Neelsen stain for acid-fast bacilli.
- Culture for *Mycobacterium tuberculosis* in Lowenstein-Jensen culture medium (may take up to 8 weeks).
- The Xpert MTB/RIF detects DNA sequences specific for *M tuberculosis* and rifampicin resistance by polymerase chain reaction in sputum in <2 hours. Research into its value in nonsputum analysis is promising.
- Histology: caseous granuloma with acid-fast bacilli is diagnostic. Granuloma without acid-fast bacilli is suggestive in the correct clinical context.

vertebral body needs to be destroyed before changes are evident; this may take up to 6 months from the time of infection.[22] Visualization is limited at the atlanto-occipital, cervicothoracic (**Fig. 1**), and lumbosacral junctions (**Fig. 2**) and the posterior elements are often poorly seen. The number of affected vertebral bodies may be underestimated and paraspinal masses or abscesses are often overlooked.[21] Plain film findings range from normal to complete loss of vertebral height (vertebra plana), a rare finding thought to be secondary to central body lysis and found more commonly in children (**Fig. 3**).[23,24] Subligamentous extension and paravertebral collections may cause scalloping and erosion (**Fig. 4**) of the vertebral bodies, and the prevertebral soft tissue associated with high cervical spondylitis may mimic a retropharyngeal collection (**Fig. 5**).[1] Thoracic paraspinal abscess may be difficult to distinguish from the descending aorta (**Fig. 6**). Examination

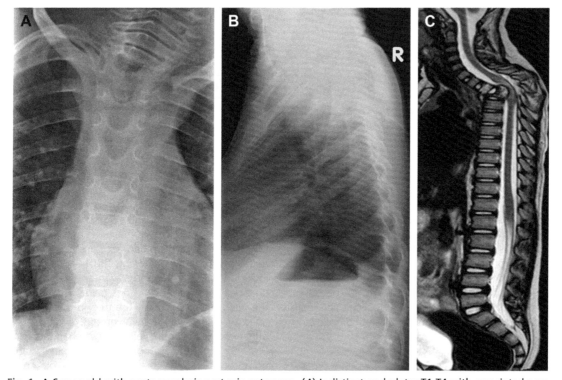

Fig. 1. A 6 year old with acute paralysis post minor trauma. (*A*) Indistinct end plates T1-T4 with associated paravertebral soft tissue mass. (*B*) Poor visualization of cervicothoracic junction with impression of gibbus. (*C*) Gibbus, cord compression, and cord signal change confirmed on MR imaging.

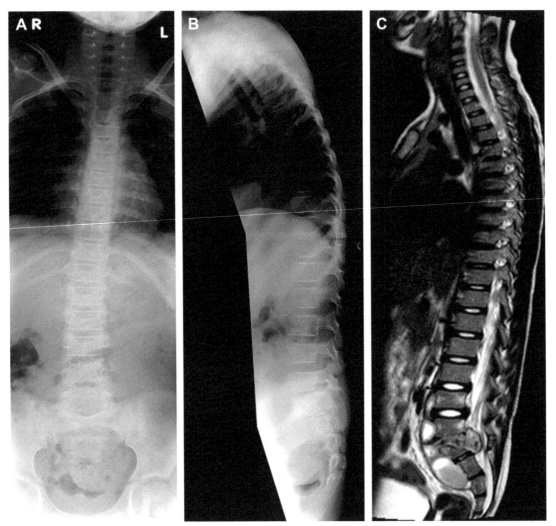

Fig. 2. A 13 year old with limp. (*A*) Vague sclerosis of S1. (*B*) Poor visualization of lumbosacral junction and erosion of anterior body of S2. (*C*) Lumbosacral spondylitis with anterior subligamentous collection elegantly demonstrated on MR imaging.

of the psoas outlines may reveal asymmetry (**Fig. 7**) and in chronic cases peripheral calcification that is pathognomonic of TB (**Fig. 8**).[25] Radiographic progression of bone destruction may continue for up to 14 months after initiation of effective chemotherapy and should not be taken as a sign of treatment failure.[26] Reactive sclerosis and periosteal reaction occur only late or following treatment.[1,24]

Computed Tomography

Computed tomography (CT) is superior to radiography in demonstrating bone involvement and soft

tissue changes and in showing subtle soft tissue calcification.[27] It is more widely available than MR imaging and may be useful in the setting of acute myelopathy. Widening the field of view to include the chest has the advantage of detecting changes of TB that may not be appreciated on the plain film, particularly the tree-in-bud appearance of early alveolar involvement, small pleural effusions, and small-volume lymphadenopathy (**Fig. 9**). Epidural soft tissue and spinal canal compromise are visible to the astute observer, although cord detail and bone edema cannot be assessed.[27] CT with multiplanar reformats reveals the anatomic extent of bone destruction,

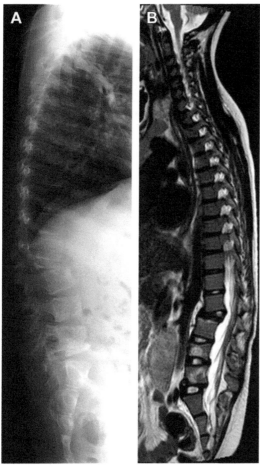

Fig. 3. A 10 year old with back pain and positive TB skin test. (*A*) Vertebra plana of L1 and L5 with anterior wedging of L3. (*B*) MR imaging confirms L1/L5 collapse and shows additional involvement of L3 and L4.

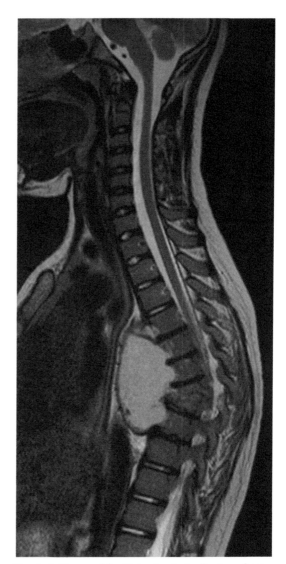

Fig. 4. A 10 year old with kyphosis. Scalloping of anterior vertebral bodies secondary to large anterior subligamentous abscess.

particularly involvement of the posterior elements leading to instability, and are invaluable for surgical planning.[26] CT-guided percutaneous biopsy and abscess drainage (**Fig. 10**) offer an alternative to the open surgical approach, although the radiation dose is of concern particularly in children.

Nuclear Medicine

Technetium-99m diphosphonate bone scans are sensitive but nonspecific in the depiction of spondylodiskitis and are poor at delineating the concomitant soft tissue extent.[28,29] Fluorodeoxyglucose PET does not provide improved specificity but demonstrates reasonable correlation with C-reactive protein as a measure of activity. It does

not perform as well as MR imaging in differentiating between TB and pyogenic spondylitis.[30]

MR Imaging

MR imaging is the imaging modality of choice in the assessment of TBS. It avoids the use of ionizing radiation and its inherent soft tissue contrast demonstrates masses, disks, and spinal cord to advantage. The entire spine should be imaged to exclude multilevel noncontiguous involvement (**Fig. 11**). A standardized protocol should be adopted (**Box 2**).

214

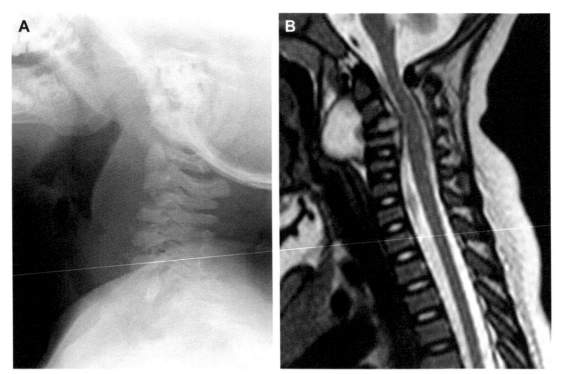

Fig. 5. A 2 year old with torticollis. (*A*) Prevertebral soft tissue swelling and destruction of C3. (*B*) MR imaging confirms anterior and posterior subligamentous collections and destruction of C3 and C4.

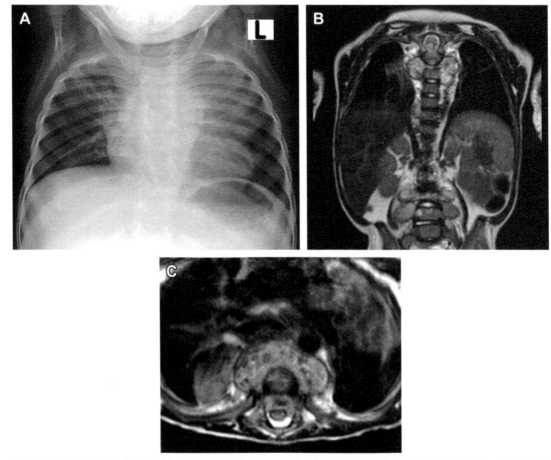

Fig. 6. A 2 year old with palpable mass. (*A*) Left paravertebral mass with left main bronchial compression and consolidation in the left upper lobe. (*B*, *C*) T2 intermediate/high signal paravertebral and epidural mass.

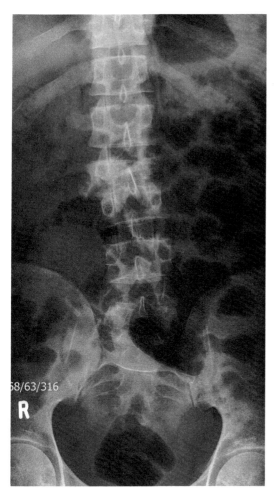

Fig. 7. A radiograph showing bulging right psoas outline in adult with TBS L2/3. Psoas abscess confirmed on MR imaging.

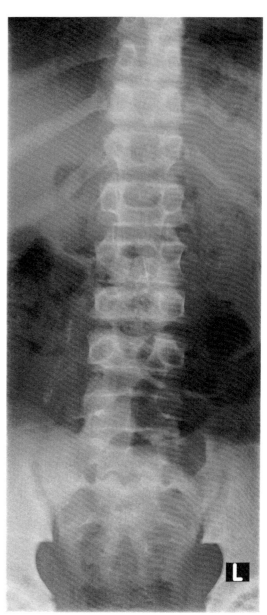

Fig. 8. A 13 year old with previous TBS and psoas collections. Narrowed L2/3 disk space, loss of height of L3/L4, and calcification of right psoas.

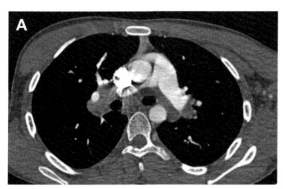
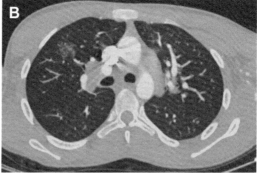

Fig. 9. A 23 year old positive for human immunodeficiency virus with TBS. Wide field of view CT demonstrating (A) hilar adenopathy on mediastinal window and (B) "tree-in-bud" appearance of early active pulmonary tuberculosis.

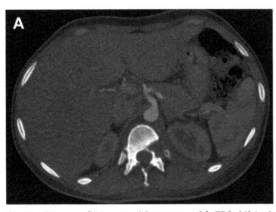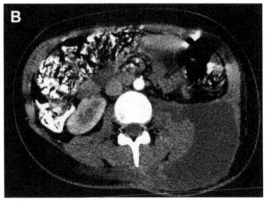

Fig. 10. CT scan of 32-year-old woman with TBS. (*A*) Lytic lesion T12 body. (*B*) Large contiguous psoas and subcutaneous abscess.

Vertebrae

Irrespective of the pattern of vertebral involvement, T1 and T2 prolongation is expected in the affected vertebral body because of replacement of normal marrow by edematous inflammatory tissue (**Fig. 12**).[27] Abnormal signal often extends into the pedicles, although the fine cortical rim of low signal seen on T1- and T2-weighted imaging is usually maintained.

Contrast enhancement in the bone depends on the pattern of destruction and may be restricted to the end plates or be more diffuse (**Fig. 13**). There is breach of the vertebral body cortex in all but the earliest of infections.

The spinous processes are invariably spared and may be helpful in defining the number of bodies involved by multilevel contiguous collapse.[31]

Disk

A great deal of emphasis has been placed on relative preservation of the intervertebral disk until late in the disease process in TBS. The MR imaging appearance at presentation in the adult and pediatric population is variable and independent of the stage and severity of disease. The disk may have normal size and signal (**Fig. 14**), be expanded with normal or increased T2 signal (**Fig. 15**), or may lose height and T2 signal (**Fig. 16**).

Soft tissues

The signal intensity of the associated epidural mass is usually intermediate to high on T2-weighted and low-intermediate on T1-weighted imaging (**Fig. 17**). Paraspinal collections return the signal of proteinaceous fluid on all pulse sequences. They occur more commonly than in pyogenic infection and may be bilateral and disproportionately larger than the degree of bone destruction. The bulk of the mass may be distant from the osteitic source (**Fig. 18**).[1,28]

In our experience the enhancement of TB abscess may be diffuse and homogeneous or, where peripheral, may be thin, thick, smooth, or nodular (**Fig. 19**). Solid enhancement, suggesting caseation without necrosis, may be difficult to distinguish from tumor (**Fig. 20**).[1,27,32]

T2-weighted coronal and axial images depict the extent of paraspinal collections and organ displacement (**Fig. 21**). Postcontrast T1 volumetric imaging allows delineation of sinuses and fistulous tracts, although in our experience the addition of postcontrast sequences does not significantly improve the specificity or positive predictive value of MR imaging.

Spinal cord

There is poor correlation between the degree of cord compression and neurology at presentation. It seems clear that the spinal canal can tolerate up to 75% loss of canal volume before symptoms occur and that the slow progression of TB allows cord accommodation.[33,34] Increased cord signal on T2-weighted imaging is associated with a worse prognosis[32] but, even where there is

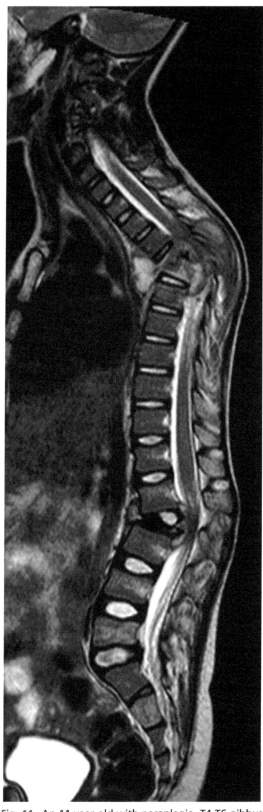

Fig. 11. An 11 year old with paraplegia. T4-T6 gibbus with intrathecal soft tissue mass causing cord compression. Also noncontiguous L2/L5 and S2 involvement.

Box 2
Suggested MR imaging protocol

- T2/FISP/FFE/GRASS coronal incorporating chest and abdomen (adenopathy, collections)
- T2 sagittal whole spine
- T2 axial through vertebral abnormality

Optional sequences

- T1 pregadolinium and postgadolinium

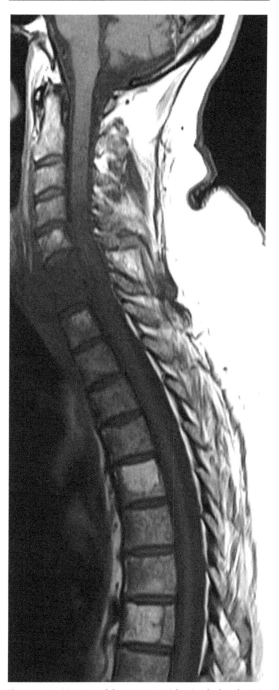

Fig. 12. A 30-year-old woman with single-level TBS. Loss of normal T1 marrow signal of C6 and C7 caused by bone edema. Note loss of disk height.

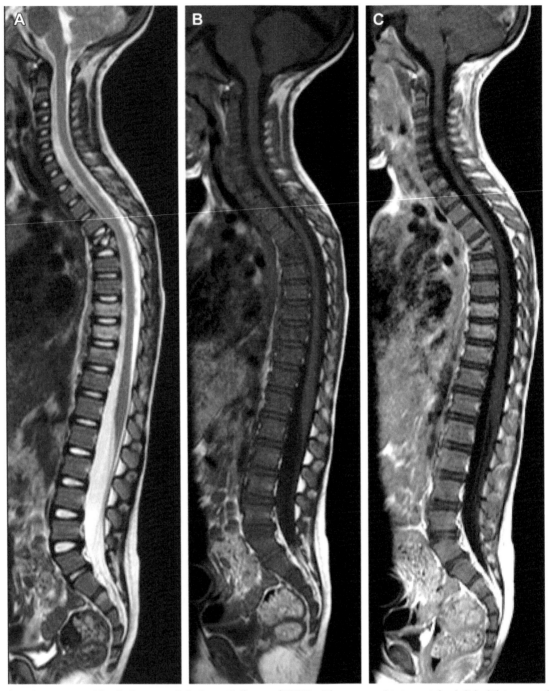

Fig. 13. A 4 year old refusing to weight bear. Collapse of T5/T6 with preserved intervertebral disk. (*A*) Increased T2-weighted signal of the bodies of T9/T10 and the superior end plates of T12 and S2 indicating bone edema. T1 sagittal pregadolinium (*B*) and postgadolinium (*C*) showing corresponding enhancement of the affected vertebral bodies.

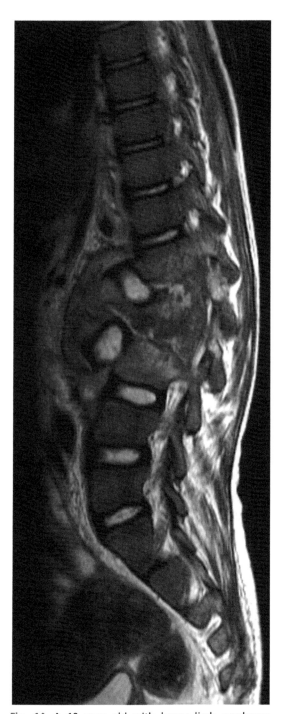

Fig. 14. A 10 year old with lower limb weakness. Expanded disks with normal signal subsumed within paraspinal abscess.

complete motor paralysis at presentation, a high percentage of patients are ambulatory posttreatment unless there is spinal arterial or venous occlusion (Fig. 22).[35]

Diffusion-Weighted Imaging

Little published data are available regarding the usefulness of diffusion-weighted imaging in the setting of spinal infection. Pui and colleagues[36] in reporting the apparent diffusion coefficient values in patients with spondylitis concluded that diffusion-weighted imaging has limited use in differentiating between TBS and pyogenic spondylitis and does not obviate biopsy.

Coronal Imaging of the Chest and Abdomen

Chest radiography reveals coexisting pulmonary TB in less than 50% of patients.[1,24,27] We recommend the inclusion of a wide field of view coronal T2 sequence to show ancillary features of TB. Low signal within nodes, lung parenchyma, and hepatic and splenic granulomas are thought to represent caseous necrosis (Fig. 23). Pericardial and pleural effusions, ascites, and fistulae return high signal.

Follow-Up MR Imaging

Sequential increase in marrow signal on T1-weighted imaging has been found to correlate well with clinical symptoms and signs.[27] Once drug sensitivity and appropriate drug compliance have been established, follow-up imaging is not recommended unless there is clinical deterioration. Progressive bone destruction and kyphosis do not imply treatment failure.

DIFFERENTIAL DIAGNOSIS

Differentiation between pyogenic spondylitis and TBS can be challenging. Non-TBS is most commonly caused by *Staphylococcus aureus*. Other causes include streptococcus, pneumococcus, enterococcus, *Escherichia coli*, salmonella, *Pseudomonas aeruginosa*, and *Klebsiella*. Distinguishing between these pathogens is not possible with imaging alone and requires laboratory testing.

Pyogenic spondylitis occurs most commonly in the lumbar spine, involving only two vertebral bodies and the intervening disk. The disk is involved early and invariably with loss of height, T2 prolongation, and enhancement centered on the disk and end plates (Fig. 24). Noncontiguous body and pedicular involvement are rare.[27,37] Epidural and paravertebral soft tissues and abscesses tend to be less well-defined. Thick

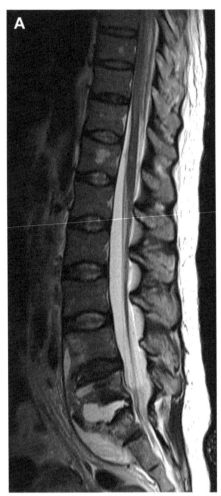

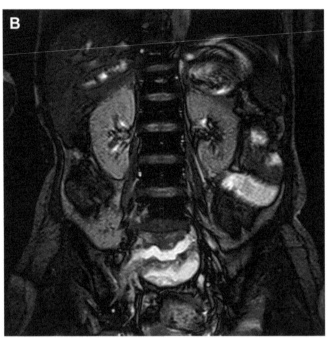

Fig. 15. A 30 year old with lower back pain. (*A*) T2 sagittal and (*B*) FISP coronal. TB spondylodiskitis with lique-faction and increased signal in the L5-S1 disk.

nodular peripheral enhancement has been described in pyogenic abscesses when compared with those found in spinal TB; however, in our experience this has poor predictive value.

Brucellosis affects the lumbar spine preferentially with anterior osteophytes (Parrot beak) described on conventional radiography. Gibbus deformity is rare and intradiscal air occurs in one-third of cases.[25,27]

Although uncommon, fungal spondylitis may be difficult to distinguish from TBS. Unlike TBS, it is seen almost exclusively in the setting of immune compromise. Both demonstrate relative disk sparing, skip lesions, and paravertebral abscesses (Fig. 25).[25,38]

Bony metastases characteristically affect multiple noncontiguous vertebral bodies and spare the disk space and the pedicles tend to be infiltrated secondarily to the posterior elements.

Lymphoma may involve a single vertebral body, pedicle, or posterior element, often with an associated paravertebral mass that demonstrates low signal on T2-weighted MR imaging (Fig. 26).

In cases where there is single body involvement or vertebra plana, Langerhans cell histiocytosis should be considered (Fig. 27).[23]

End plate signal change and disk height loss may be interpreted as type 1 Modic degeneration, although the presence of high signal in the disk on T2-weighted imaging should raise suspicion of pyogenic spondylitis or very early TBS.

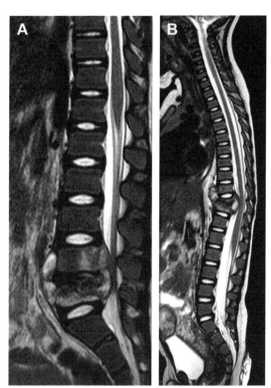

Fig. 16. (*A*) L4/L5 TBS with reduced signal of normal-sized disk. (*B*) Collapse of T10/T11; the two related disks have low signal and reduced height.

Nonspondylitic Tuberculous Myelitis

Atypical or nonosseous TB involving the cord, cauda equine, and/or the meninges is less widely reported but may be more common in human immunodeficiency virus.[15,39,40]

TB arachnoiditis is most commonly seen in the setting of tuberculous myelitis in children (72.7% of the patients with tuberculous myelitis at our institution). Adults may present with paraplegia in the absence of any signs of meningitis. Thickening, nodularity, clumping, and enhancement of the cauda equina roots on MR imaging are suggestive (**Fig. 28**).[41] Exuberant loculated enhancement throughout the thecal sac and extramedullary tuberculomas may result in meningovascular cord ischemia (**Fig. 29**).

Cord expansion and associated signal abnormality may therefore be secondary to arterial or venous infarction, or postinfectious or postinflammatory demyelination. Intramedullary tuberculomas are rare and demonstrate intermediate and/or low signal on T2-weighted imaging and rim or focal enhancement (**Fig. 30**).[41] Because cord biopsy is seldom an option, empiric treatment relies on knowledge of clinical status, cerebrospinal fluid findings, and ancillary evidence of TB.

MEDICAL MANAGEMENT OF TUBERCULOSIS

In the South African setting first-line pulmonary TB treatment is comprised of rifampicin, isoniazid, pyrazinamide, and ethambutol for 2 months followed by rifampicin and isoniazid alone for a further 4 months.

Despite a meta-analysis that concluded that 6 months treatment is sufficient for treatment of TBS,[42] in a TB endemic area extrapulmonary drug-sensitive TB (including TBS) should ideally be treated for a minimum of 12 months. In the setting of human immunodeficiency virus, 18 months of treatment is recommended. Clinical and radiographic follow-up after completion of treatment of 12 months or more is recommended.

SURGICAL INDICATIONS AND MANAGEMENT

Inability to obtain microbiologic diagnosis from microscopy, culture, or mycobacterium DNA using polymerase chain reaction may necessitate open biopsy. Corrective surgery is indicated in failed conservative treatment, progressive neurologic deficit, increase in spinal deformity, or severe pain caused by abscess. The so-called Hong Kong operation comprises radical debridement and strut grafting via an anterior approach. The procedure involves excision of the tuberculous bone until bleeding cancellous bone is exposed and creates surfaces suitable for "docking" of a strut graft (cut rib). Posterior stabilization may be required (**Fig. 31**).

SUMMARY

The prevalence of TB has increased in developing and developed countries as a consequence of the AIDS epidemic, immigration, social deprivation, and inadequate TB control and screening programs. TBS is the commonest form of skeletal TB and has characteristic imaging findings of multilevel contiguous vertebral body destruction with associated gibbus deformity. Subligamentous spread, paravertebral and epidural abscesses, cord compression, and cord edema are best evaluated with MR imaging (**Box 3**). Nonosseous spinal TB may develop in the absence of TB meningitis and is often associated with meningovascular cord ischemia. Radiologists, particularly

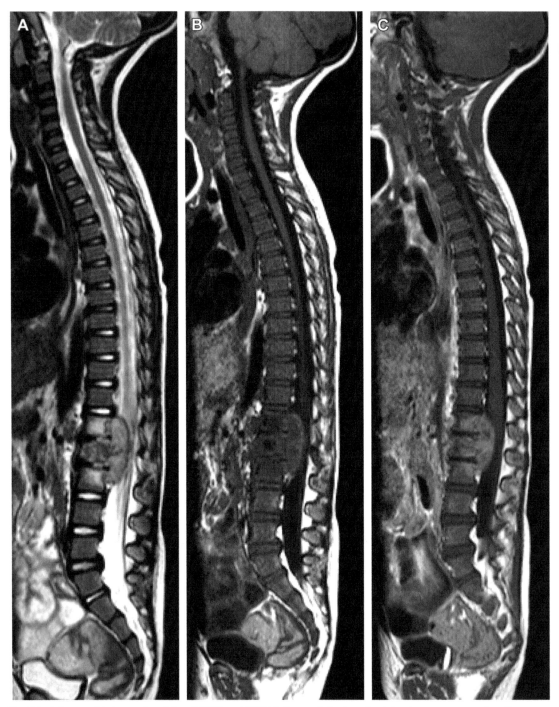

Fig. 17. A 2 year old stopped walking. (*A*) T2 and (*B*) T1 intermediate signal epidural mass compressing the conus. (*C*) The mass enhances homogeneously postcontrast.

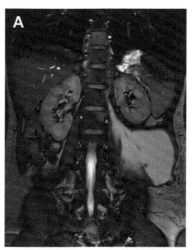

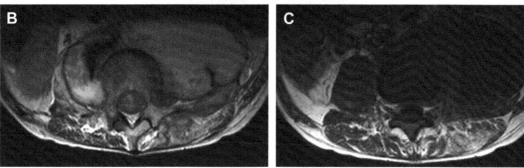

Fig. 18. A 30 year old with back pain and palpable mass. Large subcutaneous cold abscess arising from distal thoracic spondylitis. (A) FISP coronal, (B) axial T2, and (C) axial T1.

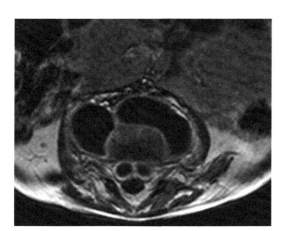

Fig. 19. A 5 year old with pulmonary TB and gibbus. T1 axial post gadolinium showing thin peripheral enhancement of paravertebral and intrathecal collections.

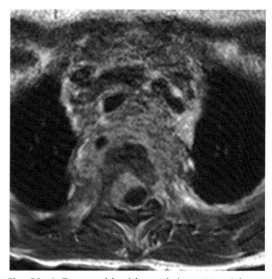

Fig. 20. A 7 year old with weak legs. T1 axial post gadolinium showing a homogeneously enhancing paravertebral collection.

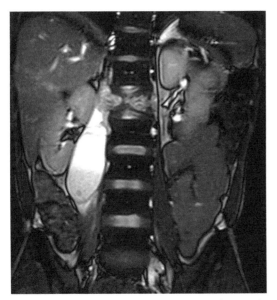

Fig. 21. A 23 year old with inability to straighten right leg. Coronal FISP showing psoas abscess displacing the right kidney superiorly.

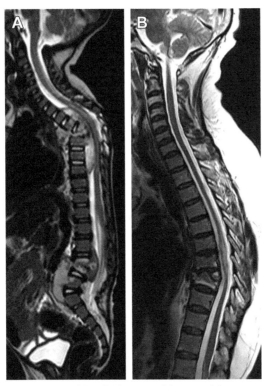

Fig. 22. (A) Child with thoracic gibbus involving T2-T7 with large epidural collection and cord edema. Noncontiguous TBS L3-S1. (B) Adult posttreatment for TBS. Counting of spinous processes proves destruction of an entire vertebral body with kyphosis and localized cord signal abnormality T8-T9.

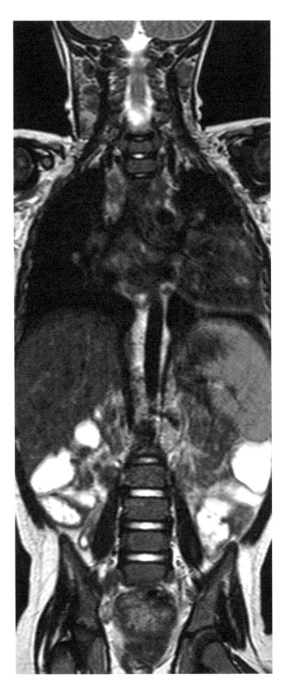

Fig. 23. A 3 year old with TBS. T2 hypointense cervical and mediastinal adenopathy and parenchymal disease of the lingula.

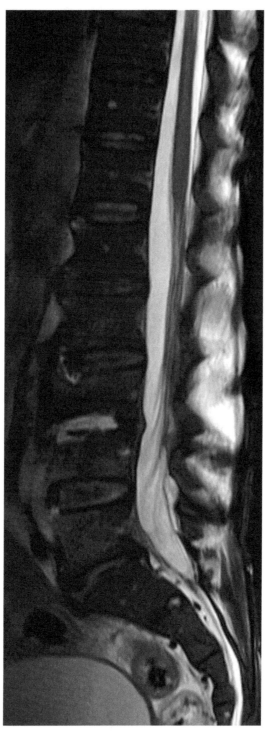

Fig. 24. A 62-year-old patient with diabetes with *Escherichia coli* septicemia and bacterial diskitis. T2 sagittal with abnormally high signal in the L3/4 disk and superior end plate of L4. Small anterior subligamentous collection.

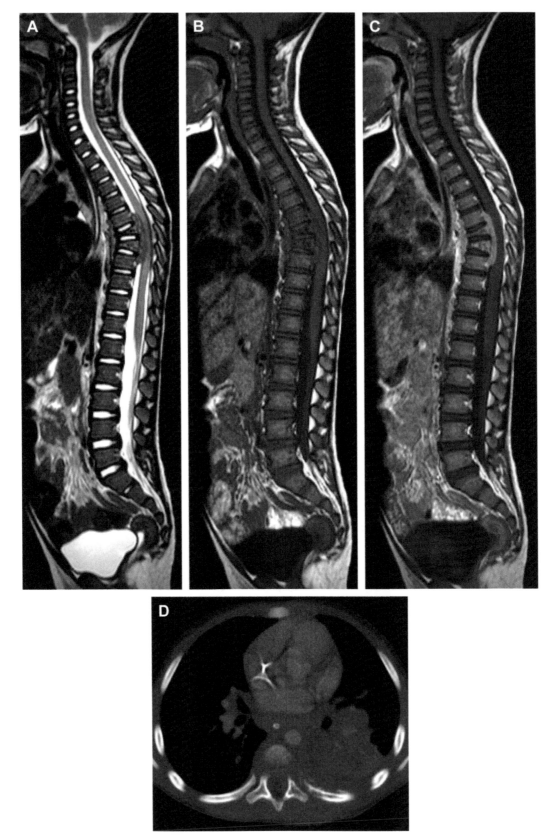

Fig. 25. A 5 year old with multiple immune deficiency and biopsy-proved disseminated *Aspergillus fumigatus*. (*A*) Anterior wedging of T8-T10 with disk preservation and profoundly T2 hypointense epidural mass compressing the cord. (*B*) Mass is isointense precontrast and (*C*) enhances homogeneously. (*D*) Paravertebral mass and rib erosion on CT.

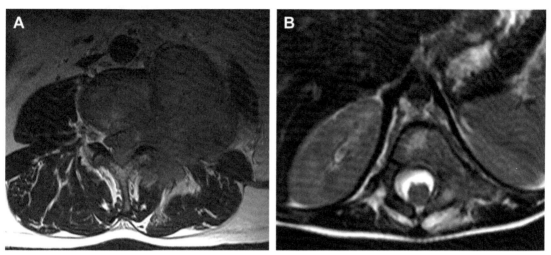

Fig. 26. (*A*) Pedicle involvement in lymphoma. Large T2 hypointense paravertebral mass with cortical destruction and neural foraminal extension. (*B*) TB, pedicle expansion without destruction of low signal cortical margin.

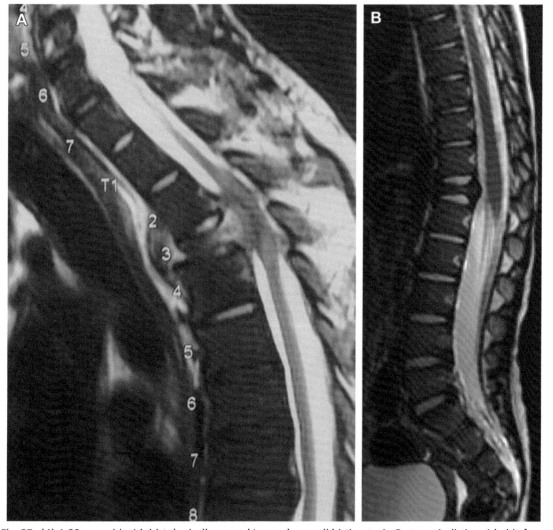

Fig. 27. (*A*) A 28 year old with histologically proved Langerhans cell histiocytosis. Features indistinguishable from TBS. (*B*) A 10 year old with Langerhans cell histiocytosis and vertebra plana.

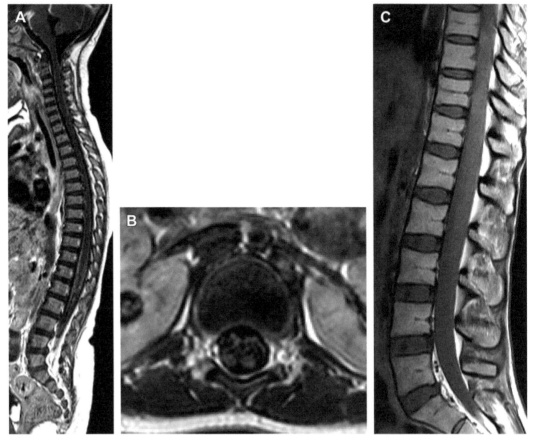

Fig. 28. A 2 year old with TB meningitis. (*A*) Sagittal and (*B*) axial postcontrast showing leptomeningeal and nerve root enhancement and nodularity. (*C*) A 33 year old with 3 months of subacute radiculomyelopathy. T1 pre-gadolinum. Increased signal in the cerebrospinal fluid in keeping with high protein.

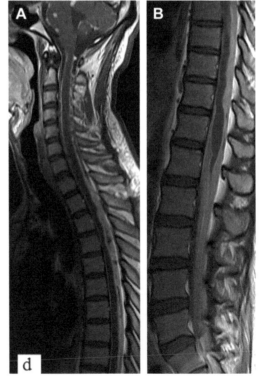

Fig. 29. A 35 year old positive for human immunodeficiency virus with (*A*) nonspondylitic TB spine and (*B*) tuber-culous enhancing granulomatous soft tissue anterior and posterior to the thoracic cord.

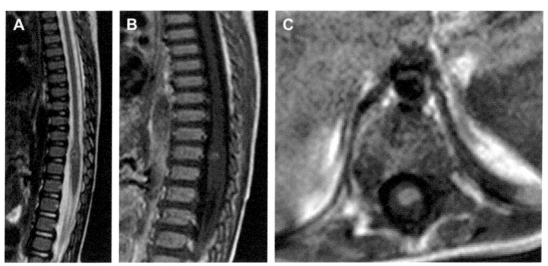

Fig. 30. A 4 year old with tuberculous myelitis. (A) Sagittal T2 hypointense intramedullary lesion. Solid enhancement postcontrast (B) sagittal and (C) axial T1.

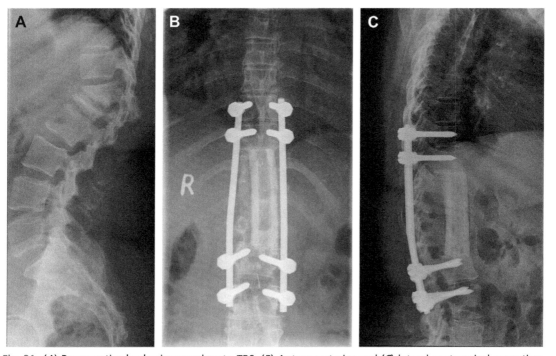

Fig. 31. (A) Preoperative kyphosis secondary to TBS. (B) Anteroposterior and (C) lateral postsurgical correction.

Box 3
Pearls

- Normal radiograph does not exclude the diagnosis; vertebral collapse may be overlooked.
- MR imaging should include the whole spine to assess for noncontiguous disease.
- Pedicular involvement does not exclude TBS.
- Disk involvement is common.
- T2 hypointense parenchymal disease and mediastinal lymphadenopathy in children and human immunodeficiency virus–positive adults indicates caseous necrosis and is suggestive of TB.

those in nonendemic areas where there may be a low index of suspicion, should be familiar with the spectrum of imaging findings, allowing early diagnosis and treatment of this potentially devastating condition.

REFERENCES

1. Prasad A, Manchanda S, Sachdev N, et al. Imaging features of pediatric musculoskeletal tuberculosis. Pediatr Radiol 2012;10:1235–49.
2. Ratcliffe JF. The arterial anatomy of the developing human dorsal and lumbar vertebral body. A microarteriographic study. J Anat 1981;133(Pt 4):625–38.
3. Ratcliffe JF. The arterial anatomy of the adult human lumbar vertebral body: a microarteriographic study. J Anat 1980;131(Pt 1):57–79.
4. Skawina A, Litwin JA, Gorczyca J, et al. The architecture of internal blood vessels in human fetal vertebral bodies. J Anat 1997;191(02):259–67.
5. Ratcliffe JF. An evaluation of the intra-osseous arterial anastomoses in the human vertebral body at different ages. A microarteriographic study. J Anat 1982;134(Pt 2):373–82.
6. Nathoo N, Caris EC, Wiener JA, et al. History of the vertebral venous plexus and the significant contributions of Breschet and Batson. Neurosurgery 2011;69:1007–14.
7. Garg RK, Somvanshi DS. Spinal tuberculosis: a review. J Spinal Cord Med 2011;34(5):440–54.
8. Pearce JM. The craniospinal venous system. Eur Neurol 2006;56(2):136–8.
9. Polley P, Dunn R. Noncontiguous spinal tuberculosis: incidence and management. Eur Spine J 2009;18(8):1096–101.
10. Gardam M, Lim S. Mycobacterial osteomyelitis and arthritis. Infect Dis Clin North Am 2005;19(4):819–30.
11. Akhtar M, Al Mana H. Pathology of tuberculosis. Tuberculosis. Heidelberg, Germany: Springer - Verlag; 2004. p. 153–9.
12. Grosset J. Mycobacterium tuberculosis in the extracellular compartment: an underestimated adversary. Antimicrob Agents Chemother 2003;47(3):833–6.
13. Kim S-S, Moon JL, Moon MS, et al. Spinal tuberculosis in children: retrospective analysis of 124 patients. Indian J Orthop 2012;46(2):150–8.
14. Yusof MI, Hassan E, Rahmat N, et al. Spinal tuberculosis: the association between pedicle involvement and anterior column damage and kyphotic deformity. Spine 2009;34(7):713–9.
15. Candy S, Chang G, Andronikou S. Acute myelopathy or cauda equina syndrome in HIV-positive adults in a tuberculosis endemic setting: MRI, clinical, and pathologic findings. AJNR Am J Neuroradiol 2014;35(8):1634–41.
16. Jain A, Sreenivasan R, Mukunth R, et al. Tubercular spondylitis in children. Indian J Orthop 2014;48(2):136–44.
17. DeSanto J, Ross JS. Spine infection/inflammation. Radiol Clin North Am 2011;49(1):105–27.
18. Jung NY, Jee WH, Ha KY, et al. Discrimination of tuberculous spondylitis from pyogenic spondylitis on MRI. Am J Roentgenol 2004;182(6):1405–10.
19. Jain AK. Tuberculosis of the spine a fresh look at an old disease. J Bone Joint Surg Br 2010;92(7):905–13.
20. Turgut M. Spinal tuberculosis (Pott's disease): its clinical presentation, surgical management, and outcome. A survey study on 694 patients. Neurosurg Rev 2001;24:8–13.
21. Nain-Ur-Rahman, Jamjoom A, Jamjoon ZA, et al. Neural arch tuberculosis: radiological features and their correlation with surgical findings. Br J Neurosurg 1997;11:32–8.
22. Desai S. Early diagnosis of spinal tuberculosis by MRI. J Bone Joint Surg Br 1994;76:863–9.
23. Sureka J, Samuel S, Keshava SN, et al. MRI in patients with tuberculous spondylitis presenting as vertebra plana: a retrospective analysis and review of literature. Clin Radiol 2013;66:e36–42.
24. Teo H, Peh W. Skeletal tuberculosis in children. Pediatr Radiol 2004;34:853–60.
25. Hong SH, Choi JY, Lee JW, et al. MR imaging assessment of the spine: infection or an imitation? Radiographics 2009;29:599–612.
26. Chapman M, Murray RO, Stoker DJ. Tuberculosis of the bones and joints. Semin Roentgenol 1979;14:266–82.
27. De Vuyst D, Vanhoenacker F, Gielen J, et al. Imaging features of musculoskeletal tuberculosis. Eur Radiol 2003;13:1809–19.
28. Go JL, Rothman S, Prosper A. Spine infections. Neuroimaging Clin N Am 2012;22:755–72.
29. Dunn R. The medical management of spinal tuberculosis. SA Orthop J 2010;9(1):37–41.

30. Lee IS, Lee JS, Kim SJ, et al. Fluorine-18-fluorodeoxyglucose positron emission tomography/computed tomography imaging in pyogenic and tuberculous spondylitis: preliminary study. J Comput Assist Tomogr 2009;33:587–92.

31. Boxer D, Pratt C, Hine A, et al. Radiological features during and after treatment of spinal tuberculosis. Br J Radiol 1992;65:476–9.

32. Andronikou S, Jadwat S, Douis H. Patterns of disease on MRI in 53 children with tuberculous spondylitis and the role of gadolinium. Pediatr Radiol 2002; 32:798–805.

33. Hoffman E, Crosier J, Cremin B. Imaging in children with spinal tuberculosis. A comparison of radiography, computed tomography and magnetic resonance imaging. J Bone Joint Surg Br 1993;75: 233–9.

34. Danchaivijitr N, Temram S, Thepmonkhol K, et al. Diagnostic accuracy of MR imaging in tuberculous spondylitis. J Med Assoc Thai 2007;90:1581–8.

35. Dunn R, Zondagh I, Candy S. Spinal tuberculosis: magnetic resonance imaging and neurological impairment. Spine 2011;36(6):469–73.

36. Pui MH, Mitha A, Rae WI, et al. Diffusion-weighted magnetic resonance imaging of spinal infection and malignancy. J Neuroimaging 2005; 15:164–70.

37. Chang MC, Hung TA, Chi-Han L. Tuberculous spondylitis and pyogenic spondylitis. Comparative magnetic resonance imaging features. Spine 2006;31: 782–8.

38. Joseffer S, Cooper P. Modern Imaging of spinal tuberculosis. J Neurosurg Spine 2005;2:145–50.

39. Thurnher MM, Post MJ, Jinkins JR. MRI of infections and neoplasms of the spine and spinal cord in 55 patients with AIDS. Neuroradiology 2000;42: 551–63.

40. Gupta RK, Gupta S, Kumar S, et al. MRI in intraspinal tuberculosis. Neuroradiology 1994;36:39–43.

41. Du Plessis J, Andronikou S, Theron S, et al. Unusual forms of spinal tuberculosis. Childs Nerv Syst 2008; 24:453–7.

42. van Loenhout-Rooyackers JH, Verbeek AL, Jutte PC. Chemotherapeutic treatment for spinal tuberculosis. Int J Tuberc Lung Dis 2002;6(3):259–65.

Spinal Brucellosis

E. Turgut Tali, MD*, A. Murat Koc, MD, A. Yusuf Oner, MD

KEYWORDS

- Spinal infection • Brucellosis • MR imaging

KEY POINTS

- Spinal involvement is common in human brucellosis.
- Osteoarticular disease and neurobrucellosis are the most common complications.
- Spinal brucellosis involves lumbar region in more than half of the cases.
- Preservation of vertebral architecture is typical.
- MR imaging is the currently the best imaging tool for diagnosis and follow-up in patients with spinal infections.

INTRODUCTION

Spinal brucellosis is a significant cause of morbidity and mortality, particularly in endemic areas. The diagnosis of spinal brucellosis is challenging but important to ensure proper treatment. Early diagnosis and treatment are crucial. Radiologic evaluations have gained importance in the diagnosis, evaluation, and treatment monitoring of all the spinal infections. Diagnosis can be made with imaging and isolation of the causative agent from blood, cerebrospinal fluid (CSF), or the lesion.

DEFINITION AND EPIDEMIOLOGY

Brucellosis (undulant fever, Malta fever) is a zoonotic disease that effects animals as the primary host (ie, camels, sheep, goats) and humans as the secondary host.[1,2] The infecting agent was first identified by Bruce in 1887 in a patient who died on the island of Malta. The disease is caused by small, nonmotile gram-negative facultative intracellular coccobacilli of the genus *Brucella*, including *Brucella melitensis*, *Brucella abortus*, *Brucella suis*, *Brucella canis*, and *Brucella ovis*, which are usually transmitted through the consumption of uncooked meat or unpasteurized dairy products.[1,2]

B. melitensis is the most common microorganism isolated in brucella spondylitis and neurobrucellosis, which is also endemic in certain parts of the world. The incidence of spinal involvement in brucellosis is 2% to 65%. Men are affected more frequently than women, which may be reflective of occupational risks such as those encountered in the stock industry, which mainly employs men.[3]

The type of skeletal involvement depends partly on the patient's age and the *Brucella* species involved. Although arthritis, bursitis, tenosynovitis, and sacroiliitis are more frequently observed in younger patients, the frequency of spondylodiscitis increases with age, and its diagnosis may be difficult because brucella spondylitis may resemble many diseases that affect the spine, such as tuberculosis, pyogenic osteomyelitis, intervertebral disc herniation, and malignancy. Brucella spondylitis presents in focal and diffuse forms, commonly in people aged 50 and 60 years of age in endemic areas.[4]

Spinal brucellosis suggests a spectrum of disease comprising infections of the numerous components of the spinal colon, including vertebral bodies (spondylitis), intervertebral discs (spondylodiscitis), facet joints (arthritis), ligaments, paraspinal soft tissues, epidural space (epidural

The authors certify that they have no conflict of interest with any financial organization regarding the material discussed in this article.

Neuroradiology Division, Department of Radiology, Gazi University School of Medicine, Besevler, Cankaya 06560, Ankara, Turkey

* Corresponding author.

E-mail address: turgut.tali@gmail.com

neuroimaging.theclinics.com

phlegmon/abscesses), meninges, and subarachnoid space and the spinal cord itself (myelitis).[5,6]

The lumbar region was noted to be the site of involvement in more than half of the cases, which was considered to be the result of its rich blood supply and higher likelihood of endplate degeneration.[7] Thoracic vertebrae are involved in 19% of the cases.[8] Cervical vertebrae are rarely affected, but this involvement is more dangerous because of potentially life-threatening complications, such as paraplegia and tetraplegia, in 1% of cases.[9,10] Multilevel involvement of brucella spondylitis has been reported to occur in 6% to 36% of cases.[7,8,11,12]

The World Health Organization estimates the worldwide incidence of new brucellosis cases to be more than 500,000 per year.[13] Brucellosis is a common cause of vertebral osteomyelitis in geographic areas in which B. melitensis is endemic (ie, the Mediterranean basin, the Middle East, Latin America).[14]

MECHANISM

Brucellosis spreads hematogenously to tissues, and almost every organ can be affected. Microorganisms at a distant septic focus reach the spine by anterograde flow through the nutrient arterioles of the vertebral bodies or by retrograde flow through the paravertebral Batson venous plexus.[9,15]

Brucella spondylitis usually begins in the superior endplate because of its rich blood supply, and causes bone destruction even in the early stages. Occasionally the inferior endplate may also be involved. The infection spreads to the remainder of the vertebral body along the medullary spaces. With the inflammatory process, the process of bone healing begins almost simultaneously, and frequently spills over in the form of anterior osteophyte, like "parrot's beak." Initially discs are spared, as they are in tuberculosis spondylitis. In the later stage, brucella spondylitis extends to the adjacent vertebrae through the intervertebral disc space. The intervertebral disc is involved as a secondary process.[7,11]

Microorganisms may leak into the CSF with the help of an inflammatory vasculitic process, resulting in spondylitis and meningitis occurring simultaneously during the acute stage masking one's symptoms over other's.[5,16] Epidural masses may accompany the whole pathologic process, sometimes causing compression of a nerve root or spinal cord, mimicking a herniated intervertebral disc.[7,17] Facet involvement (6%–35%),

intramedullary infections (1.2%–35.0%), and psoas abscess (1.2%–50.0%) are rare findings.[2,11]

Intramedullary brucella infection or abscess is rare.[18] The organism may act directly or indirectly through its endotoxins. The spinal cord or nerve root may be secondarily involved because of spondylitis, vasculitis, and arachnoiditis.[19]

Immune-mediated demyelination has been proposed to explain certain chronic forms of neurobrucellosis.[20] Impaired immune status is believed to be a risk factor for developing neurobrucellosis. Nervous system involvement in brucellosis might be from the persisting intracellular microorganisms or, perhaps, the infection triggering an immune mechanism, leading to neuropathology.[21] In an experimental animal model, the ganglioside-like molecules expressed on the surface of B. melitensis were found to induce antiganglioside membrane 1 ganglioside antibodies, resulting in flaccid limb weakness and ataxia-like symptoms.[22]

Infection triggers the immune-allergic mechanism, leading to myelopathy and/or a demyelinating state.[23] The occurrence of inflammatory central and peripheral demyelination as the pathologic manifestation of some types of neurobrucellosis, associated with inflammatory perivenular infiltration but not with histologically demonstrable organisms, strongly suggests that autoimmune mechanisms play a role in some types of neurobrucellosis.[24] This change in the spinal cord is virtually identical to that found in transverse myelitis or acute disseminated encephalomyelitis (ADEM), whereas the change that may be found in spinal roots may be identical to that found in acute inflammatory polyneuritis associated with Guillain-Barré syndrome. In these types of chronic neurobrucellosis cases, axons tend to be spared, although in severe cases, as in severe ADEM or Guillain-Barré syndrome, considerable axonal loss and associated peripheral neuroaxonal dissolution are seen.[24] It is also possible that the occurrence of a hyperergic immune response after latency from a bout of acute brucellosis is not caused by the slowed autoimmune response during a phase of chronic infection, but rather reinfection. Chronic inflammatory changes may be found in the perineurium in patients with neurobrucellosis, and adhesive arachnoiditis may develop in the subarachnoid space. Perineural inflammation may lead to dysfunction of peripheral nerves, with resulting radiculitis syndromes, especially if these inflammatory changes progress to the point of granuloma formation.[24] Recurrence of myelitis has also been reported.[25]

Chronic *Brucella* infection develops because of either the difficulties inherent in killing an intracellular parasite or inadequate treatment, rendering a potentially deleterious autoimmune response to infection, or the hosts' particular vulnerability to the immune response engendered by *Brucella* infection that have chronically infected other parts of the body or by reintroduction of infection to an already sensitized individual. Chronic brucellosis does not develop in all mistreated or untreated individuals; other host factors likely play a role in the susceptibility to chronic brucellosis, and these hosts usually harbor *Brucella* organisms in their lymphatic/reticuloendothelial system.

Brucella can cause vasculitis, either from bacterial proliferation in the vascular endothelium or from the actions of bacterial toxins. It has no predilection of size or location of vascular structure. Arterial and/or venous structures may be affected.[26,27] These vascular changes may occur in large or smaller-caliber arteries and veins, resulting in focal or multifocal arterial occlusions; venous thrombosis; lacunar, hemorrhagic, or nonhemorrhagic infarctions; mycotic aneurysm formation; subarachnoid hemorrhages from ruptured mycotic aneurysms; and subdural hemorrhages.[28–32]

CLINICAL MANIFESTATIONS

Brucellosis may appear in 4 different forms, namely acute, subacute, chronic, and relapsing.[33–35] The symptoms vary according to the site of involvement and the stage of infection.[36] The disease is characterized by a febrile illness, with severe rheumatism that occurs after an incubation period of 1 to 3 weeks.[37]

Clinically, the disease usually presents with a wide range of nonspecific clinical signs and symptoms, such as fever, malaise, profuse night sweating, weight loss, polyarthralgia, generalized myalgia, and headache. Localized back pain is the earliest and the most important symptom of brucella spondylitis, and 10% to 43% of these patients have some degree of neurologic deficit.[4,7]

Brucella is an intracellular bacterium that may remain dormant and reactivate after a variable period of clinical latency, possibly causing relapses.[38] The triggering effect of reactivation is still unknown.

Morbidity rates increase with delayed diagnosis. Neurologic complications may appear from spinal involvement of the osteoarticular disease, such as epidural abscess, radiculoneuritis, myelitis, or demyelinating neuropathy, which are the main causes of morbidity in brucellosis.[2,14,39]

DIAGNOSIS

Brucellosis has a clinical course with nonspecific symptoms and signs. Laboratory results alone are not efficient in establishing a correct diagnosis. Mildly elevated sedimentation rates and liver function enzyme levels, lowered hemoglobin levels, thrombocyte counts, and white blood cell counts are seen in most cases.

A standard tube agglutination test using smooth suspension of killed bacterial antigen may be helpful for diagnosis. Agglutination titers of 1:80 for patients without history of animal contact and 1:160 for those with a history of animal contact are considered positive findings for infection. An enzyme-linked immunosorbent assay for IgG and IgM antibodies for *Brucella* may be used, with antibody levels more than 40 arbitrary unit (AU) regarded as positive findings of infection.[37]

Definite diagnosis can be made primarily through isolation of the microorganism from blood, CSF, bone marrow or from the abscess itself. Image-guided procedures are helpful through this process, such as computed tomography (CT)–guided percutaneous biopsy. Blood culture results are not always positive for the bacteria (range, 35%–92%), because of the possible previous use of antimicrobial agents and the intermittent feature of the bacteremia.[14] Serology may help establish a diagnosis based on positive (>1:160) titers of antibodies to *Brucella* or titers greater than 1:320 on Coombs test.[14,40]

Hence, neurobrucellosis is the second most common complication of brucellosis and requires longer treatment; acute meningitis, myelitis, and myelopathy should be considered and screened for properly based on serum and CSF serology, quantitative changes in cerebrospinal CSF, and imaging studies.[39] All of this information indicates that a precise imaging study is necessary for accurate and timely diagnosis. Spinal MR imaging examination is the gold standard among all radiologic methods of diagnosis.

Plain Radiographs

Plain radiography is an easily accessible and quick method of spinal imaging. It provides information mostly about disorders of the vertebral column. It is widely used in patients with back pain, but its sensitivity is very low, especially in the early stages of brucella spondylitis. Because brucella spondylitis is a slowly progressing disorder, only one-fourth of the patients have radiologic abnormalities on admission.[6] Osteophytes, sclerosis, and osteoporosis of the vertebral body, narrowing of the intervertebral disc space are the common, nonspecific findings, usually seen in the lumbar spine, which resemble those seen in most degenerative disorders. Posterior elements are mostly preserved. No central necrosis is present and the vertebral body is mostly morphologically intact, which allows brucella spondylitis to be differentiated from tuberculous spondylitis.

Computed Tomography, Scintigraphy, and PET

CT is superior to plain radiographs in many ways. It provides detailed information about bony structures through the capability of 3-dimensional imaging. With the help of intravenous contrast agents, CT can also provide information about paraspinal soft tissue and spinal canal masses. Although it is not sensitive, and differential diagnosis from noninfectious or tumoral lesions may be difficult, it may be useful in image-guided percutaneous procedures, such as biopsy of the infected area, to confirm the diagnosis or aspiration of the paravertebral abscess.[6]

Intrathecal injection of contrast agents during CT scan or conventional myelography is contraindicated in spinal infections, because it may cause epidural infection to extend into the subarachnoid space, possibly resulting in meningitis.[41]

Bone scan with technetium 99m is rather a specific method for detecting osteomyelitis, discitis, and aseptic spinal diseases. Diffuse-form brucella spondylitis shows prominently increased extended uptake, whereas focal-form shows moderately increased uptake only in the anterior part of the vertebral body. Skeletal scintigraphy offers coarse anatomic detail and limited tissue resolution, which in turn necessitates the use of an advanced imaging method, such as MR imaging.[6,14,41]

PET scan is another alternative method that may become useful in differentiating infectious and degenerative disorders of vertebral endplates.[6,42] High 18-F Fluorodeoxyglucose (FDG)-Positron emission tomography uptake is seen in spondylitis, whereas no or low FDG uptake is evident in degenerative disorders.

MR Imaging

MR imaging is currently the best imaging tool for diagnosis and follow-up in patients with spinal infections. It has higher sensitivity and specificity[9,43] and provides more comprehensive anatomic detail, especially in the soft tissue compartments (ie, intervertebral discs, epidural space, paraspinal soft tissues, spinal canal, spinal cord, nerve roots) compared with other imaging methods.[44]

Two radiologic forms of brucella spondylitis exist: the focal form, which is limited to the anterior part of the endplate, and the diffuse form, which involves the entire vertebral body, intervertebral disc, adjacent vertebra, epidural space, meninges, and spinal cord.[44]

Osteoarticular disease is the most common complication of brucellosis. The earliest reaction in the vertebral body is the accumulation of water in the marrow, which can be detected easily by MR imaging. Even though bone marrow edema is characterized by low signal intensity on T1-weighted images (T1WI) and mainly high signal intensity on T2-weighted images (T2WI) or fluid-attenuated inversion recovery (FLAIR) images, fat-saturated short tau inversion recovery (STIR), fat-saturated T2WI, or spectroscopic inversion recovery sequences are more reliable and can detect the very early changes in the infected vertebral bodies (**Fig. 1**).

The early form of brucella spondylitis is characterized by the lysis of the anterior aspect of the superior endplate at the discovertebral junction (**Fig. 2**). Bone healing begins almost simultaneously with the inflammatory process and frequently results in the formation of an anterior osteophyte (parrot's beak), and sclerosis, but the vertebral body may remain intact through the process. Generally, the spine stabilizes itself with sclerosis and bony ankylosis in chronic brucella spondylitis, whereas vertebral collapse, angulation, and scoliosis are rare (see **Fig. 2**). Abnormal segmentation must be differentiated from bony ankylosis, because it can be mistaken due to intact architecture and anterior scalloping of vertebra bodies in brucellosis.[44] T1WI is generally helpful to show these morphologic abnormalities. Infected vertebral bodies, endplates, and involved facet joints show enhancement on fat-suppressed postcontrast T1WI.[6,11] However, it is difficult to differentiate lesions occurring in patients with known tumor, trauma, degenerative disease, prior spinal surgery, initial stages of infection, preexisting narrowed disc space, hematologic disorders, and chronic diseases. Especially in the lumbar cases, the peritoneum adjacent to the involved vertebrae may be thickened and periaortic lymph nodes enlarged.[45]

Intervertebral discs are affected only after the vertebral bodies in brucella spondylodiscitis (**Fig. 3**). Infection causes swelling of the disc, resulting in higher signal intensities in T2WI and STIR images and prominent enhancement after contrast media administration on T1WI (**Fig. 4**). These findings may also help to differentiate this condition from noninfectious degenerative diseases of the spine. A swollen intervertebral disc with a circular bulge may cause increased disc space and also may mimic disc herniation in the early stage (**Fig. 5**). The infection may result in

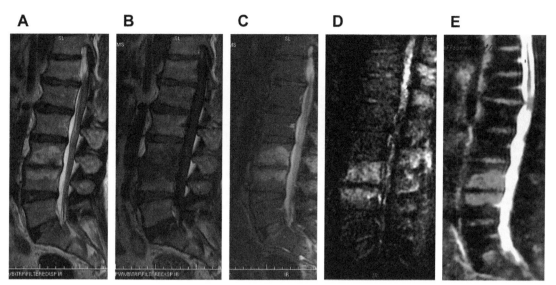

Fig. 1. Brucella spondylitis. Sagittal T2-weighted (*A*), T1-weighted (*B*), and STIR (*C*) images show involvement of L3 and L4 vertebrae and the intervertebral disc. Note the diffuse pattern of diffusion signal on sagittal diffusion-weighted imaging (*D*) and corresponding apparent diffusion coefficient map (*E*), differentiating it from the Modic type 1 degeneration with the absence of the diffusion claw sign.

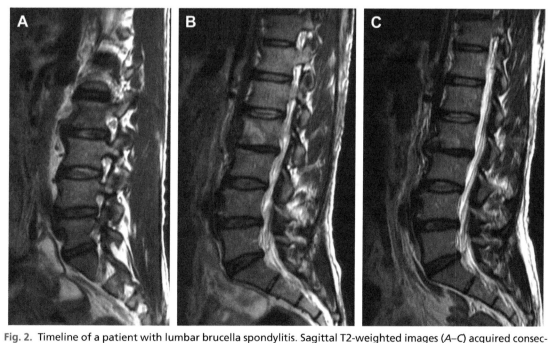

Fig. 2. Timeline of a patient with lumbar brucella spondylitis. Sagittal T2-weighted images (*A–C*) acquired consecutively within 2 years. (*A*) The earliest subtle changes are seen at the anteroinferior corner of the L2 vertebra body. A slight increase in signal intensity is the only finding at the time of examination with a sole back pain symptom. (*B*) Hyperintensity at both L2 and L3 vertebral bodies, small osteophytes at the corners, and narrowed L2–3 disc space are seen at 6-month follow-up. (*C*) Second-year evolution of the spondylitic changes, resulting in a parrot's beak–type anterior osteophyte.

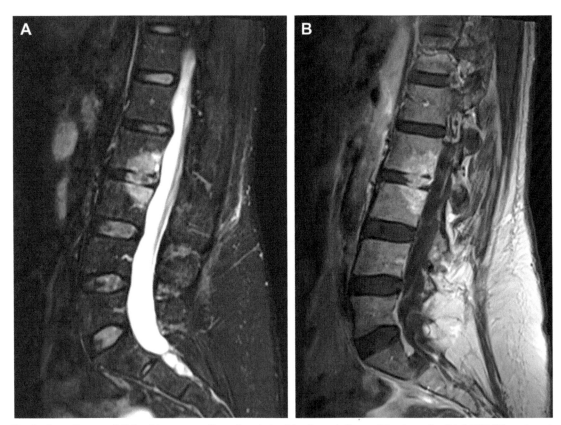

Fig. 3. Brucella spondylitis with preservation of vertebral body and disc architecture. Sagittal STIR (*A*) and postcontrast T1-weighted (*B*) images of a patient with serologically proven brucellosis show L2 and L3 vertebral bodies and the intervening disc infection. High signal intensity of prominent edema, nonanatomic enhancement of spondylitis and discitis with preservation of the vertebral body and disc architectures are seen.

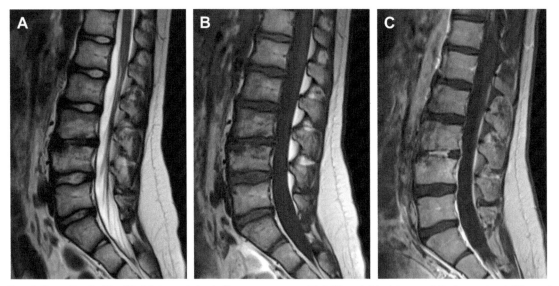

Fig. 4. Brucella discitis. L3–4 intervertebral disc space on sagittal T2-weighted image (*A*). Precontrast (*B*), and postcontrast (*C*) sagittal T1-weighted images show a slight hyperintensity at the anterior portion of the disc. Marked nonanatomic enhancement is seen on postcontrast T1WI.

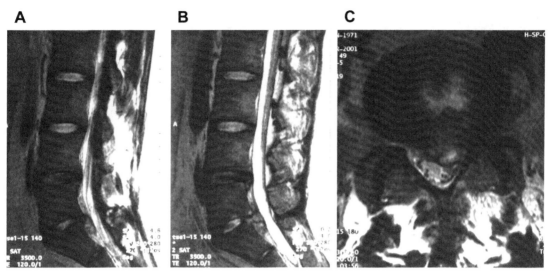

A **B** **C**

Fig. 5. Brucella discitis mimicking disc herniation. Sagittal (*A*, *B*) and axial (*C*) T2-weighted images show left paracentral-posterolateral extrusion of L5–S1 intervertebral disc. The disc shows nonanatomic high signal on T2-weighted images. Patient underwent surgery with the initial diagnosis of disc herniation, which was found to be brucella discitis at histopathology.

destruction of the entire vertebral body, leading to herniation of disc material into the endplates and causing intravertebral disc herniation. Brucellosis is characterized by a small collection of air entrapped between the disc and the affected superior endplate, referred to as "peripheral vacuum phenomenon" (up to 18%; probably caused by long-standing ischemia and avascular necrosis of the disc adjacent to the infected endplate),[46] which seems to have low signal in all MR imaging sequences. The disc space slightly decreases in later stages of the disease.[11,45] Postsurgical changes should be differentiated from discitis based on enhancement pattern; benign postsurgical changes show linear bands of enhancement in the superior and inferior aspects of the intervertebral disc that parallel the endplate margins, whereas infected discs show amorphous nonanatomic enhancement on fat-suppressed postcontrast T1WI.[41,47]

Paraspinal abscesses occur only infrequently (16%) and are of a smaller size, and paraspinal calcification is less common than in tuberculosis.[6,36,45,48,49] Increased signal intensities in paraspinal soft tissues and obliteration of muscle and fat planes, presumably by edema and/or granulation tissue, may also be seen as an accompanying paraspinal infection on T2WI. Abscess can also accompany brucella spondylitis with varying signal changes and varying ring-like contrast enhancement of the different stages.

The pathologic process may also result in spread of the infection and the granulation tissue into the epidural space with or without cord compression (**Figs. 6** and **7**). Although hematogenous spread of the infection from a distant focus is the most common mechanism of all epidural abscesses, contagious spread from adjacent spondylitis is the most common route in brucellosis.[48] Spread from paraspinal foci of suppuration and direct inoculation via penetrating trauma or neurosurgical interventions are the other causative factors. Since the hematogenous route only affects the epidural space, adjacent bony structures mostly tend to be normal. The shape of the epidural component is described as the "curtain sign" or "draped curtain sign," and can be most clearly seen on T2WI or axial fat-suppressed postcontrast T1WI because of the displacement of the posterior longitudinal ligament.[6] Since any lesion in the body of the vertebra extending to the anterior epidural space can cause the same appearance, it is not specific to the epidural abscesses. Axial and sagittal T1WI with fat suppression before and after injection of intravenous gadolinium is essential to define the extent of the disease; epidural or paraspinal abscesses and collections show enhancement.[6,11] Not only the strength of the enhancement but also the pattern of enhancement are important in diagnosis: epidural abscesses have liquid and necrotic components and show ring-type enhancement, whereas epidural phlegmons have no liquid or pus and show a diffuse-type enhancement pattern.[5,41] An epidural abscess may require emergency surgical intervention to avoid neurologic deterioration,

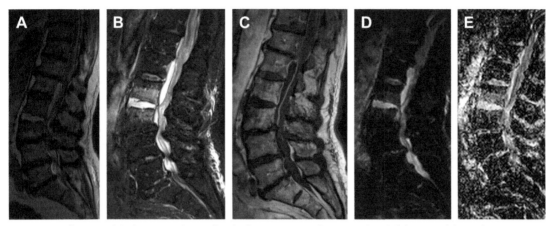

Fig. 6. Brucella spondylodiscitis with epidural abscess. Sagittal T2-weighted (*A*), STIR (*B*), and postcontrast T1-weighted (*C*) images show epidural abscess with a peripheral ring-type enhancement accompanying spondylodiscitis of L2 and L3 vertebrae. Diffusion-weighted imaging image (*D*) and corresponding apparent diffusion coefficient map (*E*) show restricted diffusion at the same level.

whereas epidural phlegmon can be treated medically with antibiotics. For this reason, an epidural abscess should be differentiated from epidural phlegmon.

Although rare, *Brucella* meningitis may cause severe complications (Fig. 8). Meningitis results in congestion and inflammation of meningeal vessels, increasing the permeability of the blood-brain

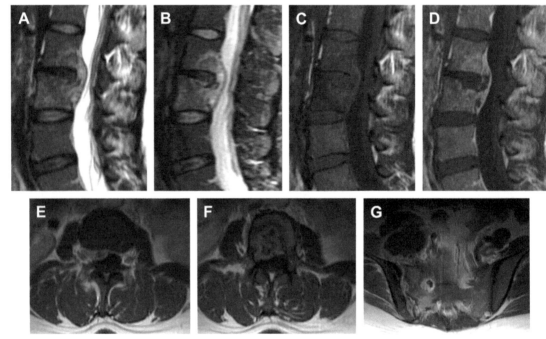

Fig. 7. Brucella spondylodiscitis with epidural abscess. Sagittal T2-weighted (*A*), STIR (*B*), precontrast (*C*), and postcontrast (*D*) images show involvement of L2 and L3 vertebrae and the intervening disc with an epidural abscess. Diffuse enhancement and extension into right neural foramen are also seen on axial postcontrast T1-weighted (*E–G*) images. Brucella sacroiliitis is also evident on the right side, together with a large psoas abscess mimicking Pott disease.

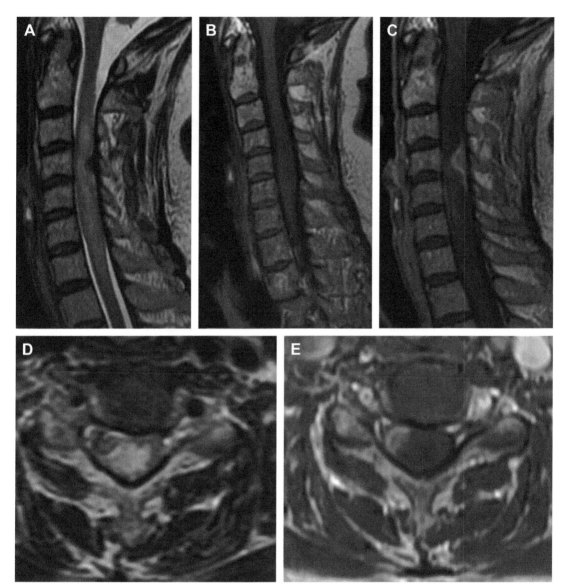

Fig. 8. Brucella myelitis and granuloma. Sagittal (A) and axial (D) T2-weighted, sagittal precontrast (B), and sagittal (C) and axial (E) postcontrast T1-weighted images show diffuse edema and swelling of the cervical spinal cord from brucella myelitis. T2-hypointense nodular granuloma located on the right side of the cord enhances markedly after contrast media administration. Accompanying pia-arachnoid–type meningitis is also noted with linear contrast enhancement.

barrier, and in distension of the subarachnoid space by exudates, causing CSF signal changes. Elevation of protein levels in the subarachnoid space and thickened meninges result in the loss of definition between the cord and CSF, loss of outline of the spinal cord, and obliteration of low signal area from increased signal of CSF and meninges on both T1WI and FLAIR images. The meningeal thickening and exudate result in blockage of CSF flow, and cause adhesions, loculations, clumping, plastering, and thickening of the roots in the lumbar region in the advanced stage. A hyperintense signal on FLAIR images is not specific for meningitis and may be seen after lumbar puncture or be associated with intracranial hypotension, subarachnoid hemorrhage, leptomeningeal metastasis, sarcoidosis, idiopathic hypertrophic spinal meningitis, Guillain-Barré syndrome, and other conditions, which should also be differentiated. Contrast media administration is mandatory when meningeal infection is suspected, because these findings may not be evident in the earliest stage. Linear and/or nodular enhancement of the meninges and nerve root sheaths are the earliest findings and may not be seen in the chronic stage. Impeded circulation of CSF by focal scarring of the meninges force CSF into the central canal of the spinal cord via the extracellular spaces. This process may cause focal cysts that eventually coalesce to form a syringomyelia. The progression of meningeal inflammation can cause the complications of vasculitis and thrombosis of the superficial pial vessels, leading to ischemia and infarction of the spinal cord.

Myelitis-myelopathy is uncommon (1.2%–30.0%).[41] Brucella may affect the spinal cord via different mechanisms, such as the infectious process of the organism, causing myelitis and spinal cord Brucella abscess; the immune-allergic mechanism, leading to a myelopathy, such as acute transverse myelitis or ADEM, and acute inflammatory polyneuritis of the roots; or the septic emboli or venous thrombosis of the Brucella vasculitis, causing myelopathy or myelitis (see Fig. 8). Presence of spinal dysraphism with persistent dermal sinus facilitates the development of intramedullary abscess. The dorsal thoracic spinal cord is the most commonly affected area, and surgery is the primary treatment method.

MR images may be normal or nonspecific during the acute phase of the myelopathy. Focal cord expansion and mild edema with ill-defined increased signal in the spinal cord on T2WI may be seen. Formation of the granuloma is a rare manifestation and may be seen as hypointense nodules on T2WI. No or mild contrast enhancement occurs in some of the cases. Prominent edema and myelitis formation with diffuse, patchy, or ring enhancement varying with the stage of the abscess formation may be seen during the subacute phase. An infected syrinx may also simulate an intramedullary abscess, particularly in the pediatric age group. It should be kept in mind that multiple sclerosis and metastasis of the spinal cord may also have the same radiologic appearance.[6] Persistent neurologic deficits are seen 70% of survivors of spinal cord abscesses, which have a mortality rate of 8% to 12%.

Diffusion-weighted imaging (DWI) is a recent technique that has been applied in the diagnosis of spondylitis. Although studies have reported the role of DWI in differentiating vertebral infections from malignancy, it was concluded that the diffusion technique is not useful because of the overlap in apparent diffusion coefficient (ADC) values.[50] Epidural abscesses also show high signal intensity in DWI and low ADC values. DWI has been shown to reveal hyperintensity in the affected vertebrae and paravertebral infectious soft tissue in acute spondylodiscitis, whereas in the chronic stage, it reveals hypointensity.[50] Spondylitis and Modic type 1 degeneration produce similar signal characteristics in the body of spinal vertebrae (ie, low signal on T1WI and high signal on T2WI) (see Fig. 1). DWI is also helpful in differentiating spondylitis from Modic type 1 degeneration. The "claw sign" refers to the highlighted borders (restricted diffusion) between normal and vascularized bone marrows in the 2 adjacent vertebrae, resembling a claw. Although normal or low signal intensity on T2WI of the intervertebral disc, favoring a degenerative process, may help exclude the diagnosis of spondylitis, higher T2 signals mostly fail to differentiate the two conditions properly. DWI might be useful in these situations; a prominent claw sign favors a diagnosis of Modic type 1 degeneration, whereas the absence of the claw (or diffuse diffusion signal) favors infection of the intervertebral disc, as stated in the study of Patel and colleagues.[51]

DIFFERENTIAL DIAGNOSIS

Diagnosis of brucella spondylitis can be made after a successful process of differentiation from other infectious/noninfectious spinal disorders. Tuberculous spondylitis is always the first disorder to be ruled out, but salmonella spondylitis, other pyogenic spondylitis, disc herniation, spondylosis, metastatic lesions, plasmacytoma, and actinomycosis should be also considered in the differential diagnosis.[11,45]

In tuberculous spondylitis, vertebral architecture is not preserved and vertebral collapse and destruction are common in the early phase of the disease, with a possible gibbus deformity, whereas in brucella spondylitis collapse and destruction of the vertebral bodies are rare and late findings. Tuberculous spondylitis also tends to have larger paraspinal/epidural abscesses and areas of paravertebral soft tissue involvement.[9] Skip lesions and multiple vertebral involvements are signs favoring tuberculous spondylitis (Fig. 9).[9,11] Facet joint involvement is rather specific to brucella spondylitis, whereas pedicle and lamina involvement is frequent in tuberculosis.[2] The involvement of posterior vertebral bodies and arches are most likely to be related with tuberculous spondylitis.[10] Paraspinal calcifications are another distinctive feature of spinal tuberculosis that can be demonstrated with radiography or CT rather than MR imaging.[9]

Degenerative disc disease is also important to differentiate from brucella spondylitis. Because in brucella spondylitis the first imaging finding is

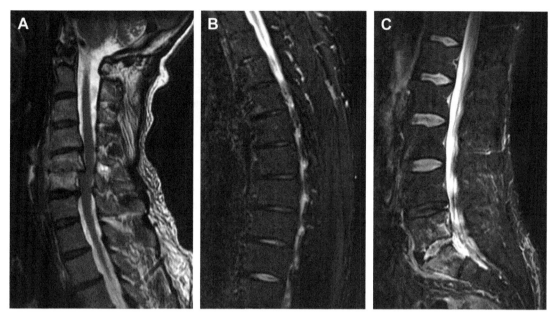

Fig. 9. Multilevel brucella spondylitis. Sagittal STIR images (*A–C*) show brucella spondylitis at C4, C5, C6, Th5, L5, and S1 vertebrae. An epidural phlegmon and discitis are also present at the lower lumbar region.

solely bone marrow edema, it is not always easy to differentiate from Modic type 1 degeneration of the vertebral endplates, which also shows inflammation and edema, but no trabecular damage or marrow change.[9] Both brucella spondylitis and Modic type 1 degeneration have high signal on T2WI and low signal on T1WI, but DWI results may appear different in terms of the "claw sign."

Although MR imaging findings suggest an infectious process in cases of brucella spondylitis, there are no characteristic features compared with other infections.[2] Pyogenic spondylitis usually has a more acute course than brucella spondylitis. Thick and irregular enhancement of the abscess wall and ill-defined paraspinal soft tissue also indicate pyogenic spondylitis.[7] Intervertebral discs are usually preserved in metastatic diseases.[45] The absence of high T2 signal in adjacent discs has also been suggested to indicate fungal spondylitis.[41]

Relative sparing of endplates and disc spaces, vertebral bodies with high signal intensity on T2WI, epidural extension, and diffuse reactive bone marrow changes simulate myeloproliferative or diffuse neoplastic disorders.

TREATMENT

Brucellosis is treated with antimicrobial agents. Treatment duration varies from 6 weeks to 6 months, and should be administered in the presence of brucella spondylitis to reduce the incidence of relapse. A synergistic or additive combination of antibiotics is required. No consensus exists about the best antimicrobial combination and treatment duration. Surgical decompression is the last resort in the management of this condition and is advised when persistent or progressive neurologic deficits occur due to compression of spinal cord or nerve roots. Patients who have rare occurence of progressive vertebral collapse or spinal instability, and who do not respond to prolonged antibiotic treatments are also potential candidates for surgery.[39,44,48]

It is well-known that brucella spondylitis is often associated with therapeutic failures.[52] Most cases of chronic brucellosis are caused by either inadequate therapy of the initial episode, focal lesions in different organs, or reactivation.

REFERENCES

1. Al-Sous MW, Bohlega S, Al-Kawi MZ, et al. Neurobrucellosis: clinical and neuroimaging correlation. AJNR Am J Neuroradiol 2004;25(3):395–401.
2. Turgut M, Turgut AT, Kosar U. Spinal brucellosis: Turkish experience based on 452 cases published during the last century. Acta Neurochir (Wien) 2006;148(10):1033–44 [discussion: 1044].
3. Ceran N, Turkoglu R, Erdem I, et al. Neurobrucellosis: clinical, diagnostic, therapeutic features and outcome. Unusual clinical presentations in an endemic region. Braz J Infect Dis 2011;15(1):52–9.

4. Raptopoulou A, Karantanas AH, Poumboulidis K, et al. Brucellar spondylodiscitis: noncontiguous multifocal involvement of the cervical, thoracic, and lumbar spine. Clin Imaging 2006;30(3):214–7.

5. Tali ET, Gultekin S. Spinal infections. Eur Radiol 2005;15(3):599–607.

6. Baleriaux DL, Neugroschl C. Spinal and spinal cord infection. Eur Radiol 2004;14(Suppl 3):E72–83.

7. Bozgeyik Z, Ozdemir H, Demirdag K, et al. Clinical and MRI findings of brucellar spondylodiscitis. Eur J Radiol 2008;67(1):153–8.

8. Chelli Bouaziz M, Ladeb MF, Chakroun M, et al. Spinal brucellosis: a review. Skeletal Radiol 2008; 37(9):785–90.

9. Hong SH, Choi JY, Lee JW, et al. MR imaging assessment of the spine: infection or an imitation? Radiographics 2009;29(2):599–612.

10. Jevtic V. Vertebral infection. Eur Radiol 2004; 14(Suppl 3):E43–52.

11. Özaksoy D, Yücesoy K, Yücesoy M, et al. Brucellar spondylitis: MRI findings. Eur Spine J 2001;10(6): 529–33.

12. Harman M, Unal O, Onbasi KT, et al. Brucellar spondylodiscitis: MRI diagnosis. Clin Imaging 2001; 25(6):421–7.

13. Aygen B, Doğanay M, Sümerkan B, et al. Clinical manifestations, complications and treatment of brucellosis: a retrospective evaluation of 480 patients. Médecine et Maladies Infectieuses 2002; 32(9):485–93. Available at: http://www.science direct.com/science/article/pii/S0399077X02004031.

14. Solera J, Lozano E, Martinez-Alfaro E, et al. Brucellar spondylitis: review of 35 cases and literature survey. Clin Infect Dis 1999;29(6):1440–9.

15. Dagirmanjian A, Schils J, McHenry MC. MR imaging of spinal infections. Magn Reson Imaging Clin N Am 1999;7(3):525–38.

16. Mousa AM, Bahar RH, Araj GF, et al. Neurological complications of brucella spondylitis. Acta Neurol Scand 1990;81(1):16–23.

17. Ozgocmen S, Ardicoglu A, Kocakoc E, et al. Para-vertebral abscess formation due to brucellosis in a patient with ankylosing spondylitis. Joint Bone Spine 2001;68(6):521–4.

18. Vajramani GV, Nagmoti MB, Patil CS. Neurobrucellosis presenting as an intra-medullary spinal cord abscess. Ann Clin Microbiol Antimicrob 2005;4:14.

19. Bashir R, Al-Kawi MZ, Harder EJ, et al. Nervous system brucellosis: diagnosis and treatment. Neurology 1985;35(11):1576–81.

20. Shakir RA, Al-Din AS, Araj GF, et al. Clinical categories of neurobrucellosis. A report on 19 cases. Brain 1987;110(Pt 1):213–23.

21. Gul HC, Erdem H, Bek S. Overview of neurobrucellosis: a pooled analysis of 187 cases. Int J Infect Dis 2009;13(6):e339–43.

22. Watanabe K, Kim S, Nishiguchi M, et al. Brucella melitensis infection associated with Guillain-Barre syndrome through molecular mimicry of host structures. FEMS Immunol Med Microbiol 2005;45(2):121–7.

23. Seidel G, Pardo CA, Newman-Toker D, et al. Neurobrucellosis presenting as leukoencephalopathy: the role of cytotoxic T lymphocytes. Arch Pathol Lab Med 2003;127(9):e374–7.

24. Robert S, Rust J. Brucellosis. 2004. Available at: http://emedicine.medscape.com/article/213430. Accessed October 7, 2014.

25. Krishnan C, Kaplin AI, Graber JS, et al. Recurrent transverse myelitis following neurobrucellosis: immunologic features and beneficial response to immunosuppression. J Neurovirol 2005;11(2):225–31.

26. Milionis H, Christou L, Elisaf M. Cutaneous manifestations in brucellosis: case report and review of the literature. Infection 2000;28(2):124–6.

27. Aguado JM, Barros C, Gomez Garces JL, et al. Infective aortitis due to Brucella melitensis. Scand J Infect Dis 1987;19(4):483–4.

28. al Deeb SM, Yaqub BA, Sharif HS, et al. Neurobrucellosis: clinical characteristics, diagnosis, and outcome. Neurology 1989;39(4):498–501.

29. Adaletli I, Albayram S, Gurses B, et al. Vasculopathic changes in the cerebral arterial system with neurobrucellosis. AJNR Am J Neuroradiol 2006;27(2):384–6.

30. Hernandez MA, Anciones B, Frank A, et al. Neurobrucellosis and cerebral vasculitis. Neurologia 1988;3(6):241–3.

31. Martin Escudero JC, Gil Gonzalez MI, Aparicio Blanco M. Intracranial hypertension and subarachnoid hemorrhage: the forms of presentation of neurobrucellosis. An Med Interna 1990;7(7):358–60.

32. Zaidan R, Al Tahan AR. Cerebral venous thrombosis: a new manifestation of neurobrucellosis. Clin Infect Dis 1999;28(2):399–400.

33. Edward JY. Brucella species. In: Mandell GL, Bennett JE, Dolin R, editors. Principles and practice of infectious diseases. 6th edition. Philadelphia: Churchill Livingstone; 2005. p. 2669–72.

34. Doganay M, Meşe-Alp E, Bruselloz. In: Topcu AW, Söyletir G, Doganay M, editors. İnfeksiyon hastalıkları ve mikrobiyolojisi. 3rd edition. Istanbul (Turkey): Nobel Tıp Kitabevleri; 2008. p. 879–909.

35. Gotuzzo E, Celillo E. Brucella. In: Gorbach SI, Bartlett JG, Blacklow NR, editors. Infectious diseases. Philadelphia: Harcourt Brace Jovanovich Inc; 1992. p. 1513–8.

36. Rajapakse CN. Bacterial infections: osteoarticular brucellosis. Baillieres Clin Rheumatol 1995;9(1): 161–77.

37. Gokhale YA, Ambardekar AG, Bhasin A, et al. Brucella spondylitis and sacroiliitis in the general population in Mumbai. J Assoc Physicians India 2003;51:659–66.

38. Solera J, Martinez-Alfaro E, Espinosa A, et al. Multivariate model for predicting relapse in human brucellosis. J Infect 1998;36(1):85–92.

39. Tur BS, Suldur N, Ataman S, et al. Brucellar spondylitis: a rare cause of spinal cord compression. Spinal Cord 2004;42(5):321–4.

40. Buzgan T, Karahocagil MK, Irmak H, et al. Clinical manifestations and complications in 1028 cases of brucellosis: a retrospective evaluation and review of the literature. Int J Infect Dis 2010;14(6):e469–78.

41. Lury K, Smith JK, Castillo M. Imaging of spinal infections. Semin Roentgenol 2006;41(4):363–79.

42. Stumpe KD, Zanetti M, Weishaupt D, et al. FDG positron emission tomography for differentiation of degenerative and infectious endplate abnormalities in the lumbar spine detected on MR imaging. AJR Am J Roentgenol 2002;179(5):1151–7.

43. Ledermann HP, Schweitzer ME, Morrison WB, et al. MR imaging findings in spinal infections: rules or myths? Radiology 2003;228(2):506–14.

44. Hantzidis P, Papadopoulos A, Kalabakos C, et al. Brucella cervical spondylitis complicated by spinal cord compression: a case report. Cases J 2009;2:6698.

45. Tali ET. Spinal infections. Eur J Radiol 2004;50(2):120–33.

46. Tekkok IH, Berker M, Ozcan OE, et al. Brucellosis of the spine. Neurosurgery 1993;33(5):838–44.

47. Longo M, Granata F, Ricciardi K, et al. Contrast-enhanced MR imaging with fat suppression in adult-onset septic spondylodiscitis. Eur Radiol 2003;13(3):626–37.

48. Kose S, Senger SS, Cavdar G, et al. Case report on the development of a brucellosis-related epidural abscess. J Infect Dev Ctries 2011;5(5):403–5.

49. Sharif HS, Aideyan OA, Clark DC, et al. Brucellar and tuberculous spondylitis: comparative imaging features. Radiology 1989;171(2):419–25.

50. Oztekin O, Calli C, Adibelli Z, et al. Brucellar spondylodiscitis: magnetic resonance imaging features with conventional sequences and diffusion-weighted imaging. Radiol Med 2010;115(5):794–803.

51. Patel KB, Poplawski MM, Pawha PS, et al. Diffusion-weighted MRI "claw sign" improves differentiation of infectious from degenerative modic type 1 signal changes of the spine. AJNR Am J Neuroradiol 2014;35(8):1647–52.

52. Bosilkovski M, Krteva L, Caparoska S, et al. Osteoarticular involvement in brucellosis: study of 196 cases in the Republic of Macedonia. Croat Med J 2004;45(6):727–33.

Viral Infection of the Spinal Cord and Roots

Hajime Yokota, MD, PhD[a,b,*], Kei Yamada, MD, PhD[a]

KEYWORDS

• Spinal cord • Myelopathy • Radiculopathy • MR imaging

KEY POINTS

- Patients with viral infections of the spinal cord and roots present with various clinical and radiologic manifestations that are induced by either direct injury from infection and/or indirect injury via the autoimmune processes.
- A combination of clinical information, including the clinical course, symptoms, laboratory data, and imaging, is essential for making a correct diagnosis.
- The time course and anatomic distribution are particularly important for differential diagnosis.

Myelitis and radiculitis are characterized by inflammatory processes of the spinal cord and nerve roots, respectively. Many different types of viruses can affect the spinal cord and roots, and infants to elderly patients are affected. Viral infection of the spinal cord is rare and is thus frequently misdiagnosed. Viral infection can directly destroy the cells of the spinal cord and roots or can cause demyelination and inflammation from abnormal immune responses of the host. The latter is usually called myelopathy, rather than myelitis.

Very few tools allow absolute diagnosis of myelopathy and radiculopathy.[1–4] Almost all myelopathies and radiculopathies are therefore included in differential diagnosis for viral infections (Box 1). To reach a correct diagnosis, a detailed clinical history, neurologic examination, laboratory tests, and imaging examination are necessary.

The complicated tract decussation of the spinal cord and roots can complicate the interpretation of neurologic examinations. Symptoms, such as paraplegia, quadriplegia, gait disturbance, sensory impairment, and bowel or bladder dysfunction, imply the presence of myelopathy. Myelitis is possible when these symptoms occur acutely and when one excludes the possibility of a compressive spinal cord lesion, neoplasm, or vascular lesion including infarction and hemorrhage.

Radiculopathy sometimes shares common neurologic symptoms with myelopathy. Important points to consider for differentiation are the tendon reflex and the type of paralysis. Radiculopathy can present with tendon hyporeflexia and flaccid paralysis, whereas myelopathy can show tendon hyperreflexia and spastic paralysis. Muscle atrophy is common in radiculopathy but less so in myelopathy. However, myelopathy and radiculopathy can occur simultaneously because viral infection can occur in the spinal cord and roots at the same time.

The speed of onset and clinical course are the most important types of information needed for diagnosing neurologic disorders. Most vascular lesions have a sudden onset, and the symptoms reach completion immediately. Demyelination, including that seen in multiple sclerosis or neuromyelitis optica, is polyphasic. Neoplasms generally have a progressive course. Degenerative and

Disclosures: None.
[a] Department of Radiology, Graduate School of Medical Science, Kyoto Prefectural University of Medicine, Kyoto, Japan; [b] Department of Diagnostic Radiology and Radiation Oncology, Graduate School of Medicine, Chiba University, Chiba, Japan
* Correspondence author. Department of Radiology, Kyoto Prefectural University of Medicine, 465 Kajii-cho, Kamigyo-ku, Kyoto 602-8566, Japan.
E-mail address: hjmykt@koto.kpu-m.ac.jp

Neuroimag Clin N Am 25 (2015) 247–258
http://dx.doi.org/10.1016/j.nic.2015.01.005

Box 1
Differential diagnosis for viral infection of the spinal cord and roots

1. Infectious myelitis
   i. Viral myelitis
      a. Varicella zoster virus
      b. Herpes simplex virus
      c. Cytomegalovirus
      d. Epstein-Barr virus
      e. Enterovirus (poliovirus, enterovirus 71, coxsackievirus, echovirus)
      f. Rabies virus
      g. Flavivirus (Japanese encephalitis), West Nile virus
      h. Human T-lymphotropic virus 1
      i. Human immunodeficiency virus
   ii. Bacterial, fungal, and parasite myelitis
      a. Mycoplasma
      b. Lyme disease
      c. Pyogenic myelitis
      d. Tuberculosis
      e. Syphilis
      f. Fungi and parasites
2. Noninfectious myelitis/myelopathy
      a. Postinfection, postvaccination (related to measles, rubella, mumps, influenza, mycoplasma, streptococcus pneumonia, and so forth)
      b. Multiple sclerosis and acute disseminated encephalomyelitis
      c. Autoimmune disorders (systemic lupus erythematosus, Sjögren syndrome, antineutrophil cytoplasmic autoantibody–related vascultiis, atopic myelitis, and so forth)
      d. Sarcoidosis
      e. Behçet's syndrome
      f. Paraneoplastic syndrome

Acute disseminated encephalomyelitis (ADEM), Guillain-Barré syndrome (GBS), and acute transverse myelitis (ATM) often appear 7 to 10 days after the onset of infection. Chronic and progressive myelitis can be caused by retroviruses, such as human T-lymphotropic virus type 1 (HTLV-1), causing HTLV-1–associated myelopathy (HAM). Some patients with human immunodeficiency virus (HIV) may also present with myelopathy.

Examination of blood and cerebrospinal fluid (CSF) often leads to a final diagnosis, but the sensitivity is often low. Blood tests should look for autoimmune antibodies, which indicate autoimmune disorders; angiotensin-converting enzyme, which indicates sarcoidosis; and IgE, which indicates parasite infection and atopic myelitis. CSF examination can be performed to look for antibodies, and polymerase chain reaction (PCR) can detect the viral genome. CSF should be evaluated for oligoclonal bands to diagnose multiple sclerosis. PCR for viral DNA is sometimes negative even though antibodies are detectable. The ability to directly identify the virus strongly depends on the timing of CSF sampling. Electrophysiologic tests are often useful for evaluating peripheral nerves, and this technique can prove the presence of radiculopathy and distinguish axonal injury from demyelination of the nerves.

Magnetic resonance (MR) imaging is an essential tool in diagnosis. However, because imaging findings are often nonspecific, consideration of a combination of the previously mentioned diagnostic procedures, including the clinical course, symptoms, and laboratory data, is necessary for making a correct diagnosis. One of the most important roles of MR imaging is to exclude other disorders, especially compressive cord lesions and vascular lesions.

Sagittal and axial image acquisitions are fundamentally important. Sagittal images provide an overview of the spinal cord and the roots. Transaxial images better depict detailed structures. For instance, because of decreased partial volume averaging for axially oriented lesions, the presence of contrast enhancement of the cord and the cauda equina is often more apparent on transaxial slices (Fig. 1). T2-weighted imaging is one of the most important sequences for detecting lesions and evaluating their distribution. Precontrast- and postcontrast-enhanced T1-weighted images are also essential for detecting abnormal vasculature and evaluating activity of the lesions. Detailed comparison between precontrast and postcontrast T1-weighted images is especially needed for the cauda equina because enhancement of this structure is sometimes vague. The number of lesions, length of the involved cord, presence or

congenital diseases are usually slowly progressive, although degeneration can fluctuate. Inflammation including viral infections shows a varied course, ranging from acute to chronic. Acute myelitis and radiculitis are frequently associated with fever, fatigue, and skin rash. Herpes viruses, such as varicella zoster virus (VZV), cytomegalovirus (CMV), Epstein-Barr virus, and herpes simplex virus, and enteroviruses including poliovirus and enterovirus 71, can show acute onset and progression of symptoms.

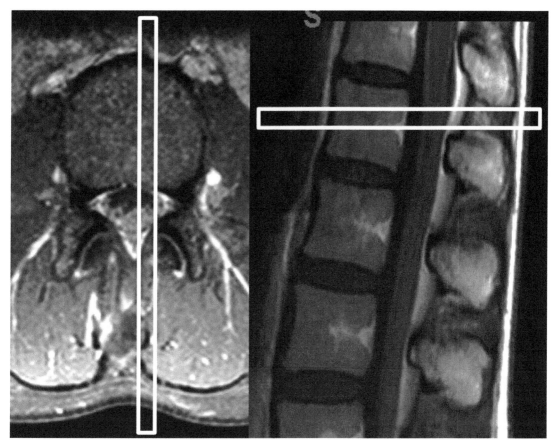

Fig. 1. The cauda equina exhibits contrast enhancement on transaxial (*left*) and sagittal (*right*) views, but it is much easier to see on the transaxial image. This is because of partial volume averaging of the thin structure running in the axial orientation, making visualization more optimal on transaxial images.

absence of atrophy or swelling, and anatomic distribution of signal abnormalities are important features to interpret.[5] Some diseases present with characteristic imaging findings. For example, VZV tends to injure the dorsal column, whereas poliovirus tends to injure the frontal horns.

In the following sections are summarized the myelopathy and radiculopathy caused by different viruses. The cases described are divided into three categories: (1) acute myelitis and radiculitis, (2) postinfectious myelopathy and radiculopathy, and (3) chronic myelopathy.

ACUTE MYELITIS AND RADICULITIS
Varicella Zoster Virus

VZV is a relatively well-documented cause of viral myelitis (**Figs. 2** and **3**). VZV usually causes encephalomyelitis, and exclusive involvement of the spinal cord has rarely been documented. Damage to the spinal cord is induced by VZV infection, excessive immune response, and vasculitis. Clinical diagnosis of VZV myelitis is usually established by the typical

time course between occurrence of a skin rash and subsequent spinal cord symptoms. Myelitis occurs after a few days to weeks from the onset of the skin rash.[6] Additional tests may be necessary, especially in immunocompromised patients who may lack the preceding skin rash, although the sensitivity of such tests may not be sufficiently high. Quick tests of choice include PCR and/or direct detection with fluorescent antibodies, the results of which can be obtained within a few hours. Viral culture, however, requires prolonged incubation and sensitivity that is lower than that of PCR. Antibodies to VZV in the CSF may be useful for diagnosing VZV myelitis. Serum antibodies, however, are often detected in patients with a history of prior infection of VZV and are thus nonspecific. Laterality between skin rash and neurologic symptoms usually matches because VZV reaches the spinal cord via the dorsal nerve root. Unilateral or asymmetric motor/sensory disturbances and bowel/bladder dysfunctions can occur.

Pathologic evaluation often shows that the entry portion of the dorsal root and the posterior column

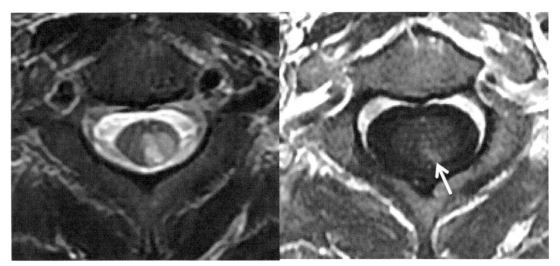

Fig. 2. VZV myelitis in a 30-year-old man with numbness of his left side. T2-weighted and contrast-enhanced T1-weighted images show involvement of the dorsal column and posterior horn (*arrow*). (*Courtesy of* A. Yagishita, MD, Y. Nakata, MD, Tokyo Metropolitan Neurological Hospital, Tokyo, Japan.)

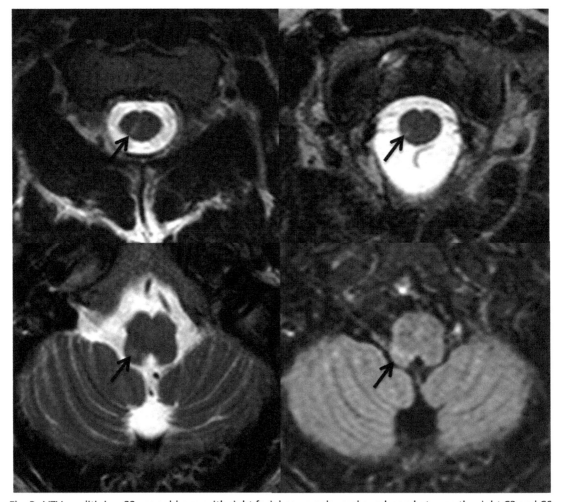

Fig. 3. VZV myelitis in a 32-year-old man with right facial nerve palsy and numbness between the right C3 and C6. Abnormal signals involving the dorsal column that reached the level of the medulla oblongata are seen (*arrows*). This long cord lesion is observed along the dorsal column–lemniscal tract involving the sensory spinal tract.

are strongly damaged. Vertical extension along the cord is also often observed.[6] The level of the skin rash and the level of the spinal cord lesions usually match on pathologic examinations, although some discrepancy can occur.

MR imaging can show pathologic changes with preferential involvement of the ipsilateral dorsal column and posterior horn.[7,8] Lesions may show enhancement in the acute phase. These imaging findings are characteristic and useful for making the diagnosis. VZV myelitis sometimes presents in long segments.[7,9] Radiculitis has also been reported.

Poliovirus

Acute poliovirus infection is typically characterized by flaccid paralysis, and is a typical pathogen causing anterior horn myelitis (**Fig. 4**).[10,11] Vaccination can dramatically reduce the incidence of poliomyelitis. New cases of poliomyelitis that we encounter are often related to live vaccination, although its incidence is now extremely low, because the inactivated vaccine is becoming more popular.

Patients with a previous history of poliomyelitis sometimes have new or progressive disability including muscle weakness, numbness, and pain that occurs 10 to 50 years after the initial onset of myelitis.[12–14] This condition is called postpolio syndrome (PPS) and is not a recurrence of poliomyelitis but a secondary disorder. Even light exercise can overload muscles already damaged by poliomyelitis and cause secondary nerve and muscle degeneration. In addition, aging changes and muscle disuse can accelerate the weakness.

The incidence of PPS is 40% to 60% in patients with previous poliomyelitis. PPS has no pathognomonic clinical findings. Laboratory tests, electromyography, and muscle biopsy are mainly used to exclude other diseases.

On MR imaging, acute-phase poliomyelitis is characterized by localized unilateral or bilateral signal abnormalities in the anterior horn. These signal changes often remain until the chronic phase. No specific imaging sign for PPS exists, and MR imaging cannot distinguish patients with previous poliomyelitis with PPS from those without symptoms of PPS. MR imaging for PPS is therefore used to exclude other causes of progressive disability.

Enterovirus 71

Acute flaccid paralysis is not specific for poliovirus infection but can be caused by various other viruses, including coxsackievirus, Japanese encephalitis virus, echovirus, or enterovirus.[15–18] This condition is known as polio-like syndrome and generally has better prognosis than poliomyelitis.

Enterovirus 71 is a cause of hand-foot-and-mouth disease (**Fig. 5**). Acute flaccid paralysis caused by enterovirus 71 radiculomyelitis has been recently documented in young children. Clinical symptoms are similar to poliomyelitis, but enterovirus 71 tends to present with myoclonus, tremor, or ataxia. The diagnosis can be made by virus isolation, PCR of CSF, or a throat swab. The sensitivity of PCR is generally superior to virus isolation using cell culture. The serology test is limited for routine diagnosis of enterovirus infections because the method is not feasible to test multiple live viral antigens and is relatively insensitive. On MR imaging, the anterior horns and ventral nerve roots are predominantly involved, and dorsal roots are usually spared.[3,15] These imaging findings closely reflect the clinical symptoms. Enterovirus can also cause rhombencephalitis.[16,17]

POSTINFECTIOUS MYELOPATHY AND RADICULOPATHY
Acute Disseminated Encephalomyelitis

ADEM is a disease with disseminated demyelination and inflammation in the brain, spinal cord, and optic nerves (**Fig. 6**). Viral infection or vaccination can cause ADEM from an abnormal autoimmune reaction. One proposed mechanism is the cross-reactivity of antibodies to infecting pathogens with normal myelin proteins. ADEM is predominantly seen in children and is rarely seen in the elderly. Idiopathic ADEM is common in adults.[19–21]

About 50% to 75% of children with ADEM have febrile illness within the 4 weeks before the onset

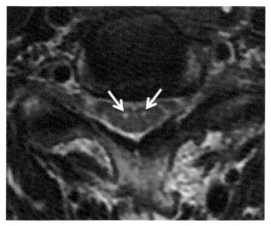

Fig. 4. Previous poliomyelitis in a 50-year-old man with progressive muscle weakness. He suffered from poliomyelitis in childhood. The bilateral anterior horns show hyperintensity on this T2-weighted image (*arrows*).

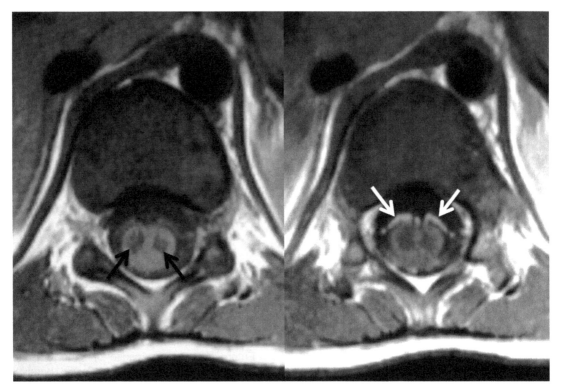

Fig. 5. Enterovirus 71 radiculomyelitis with acute flaccid paralysis. The bilateral anterior horns and ventral nerve roots are involved (*arrows*). (*Adapted from* Chen CY, Chang YC, Huang CC, et al. Acute flaccid paralysis in infants and young children with enterovirus 71 infection: MR imaging findings and clinical correlates. AJNR Am J Neuroradiol 2001;22(1):203.)

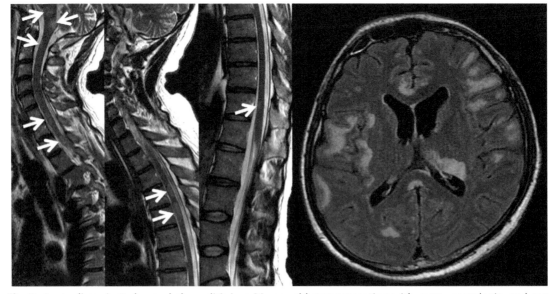

Fig. 6. Acute disseminated encephalomyelitis in a 36-year-old man presenting with coma, paraplegia, and convulsions after antecedent infection. Disseminated lesions in the spinal cord and brain are visible (*arrows*). The clinical presentation of multiple sclerosis is quite different from this case because patients with multiple sclerosis rarely present with coma.

of neurologic symptoms. Measles, mumps, rubella, varicella, and zoster are likely to be recognized as antecedent infections because they are associated with characteristic clinical findings including skin rash. In cases caused by a vaccine, ADEM typically develops 10 to 14 days after vaccination.

Typical clinical presentations include fever, meningeal irritation, leukocytosis, and pleocytosis. Disturbances in consciousness, ranging from drowsiness to coma, convulsions, and nuchal rigidity, can also develop in these patients. Respiratory disturbances are also seen in 11% to 16% of cases.

Spinal lesions can cause paraplegia, quadriplegia, tendon hyperreflexia, morbid reflection, segmental sensory impairment, and bowel or bladder dysfunction. ADEM is diagnosed based on clinical and imaging findings because no specific confirmatory biomarkers currently exist. Cases with antecedent infection or vaccination are relatively easy to diagnose, whereas reaching a solid conclusion in cases without known causes is much more difficult. ADEM is fundamentally monophasic, although some cases develop multiple sclerosis.

On imaging, spinal cord lesions show either long cord distribution or multiple discontinuous lesions and are commonly associated with swelling and contrast enhancement.[21] Differential diagnosis of long cord lesions includes ATM of various causes, whereas the latter includes multiple sclerosis. Some important points should be considered for differentiation. Almost all cases of ADEM show encephalopathy with multifocal neurologic deficits and imaging abnormalities in the brain. Discrepancies between clinical and imaging findings are often present.[22] Imaging findings typically tend to evolve with the clinical course, but lesions can often appear after improvement in the clinical symptoms. Enhancement of the nerve roots may be detected, implying demyelination of the peripheral nerves.[23]

Guillain-Barré Syndrome

GBS is a counterpart to ADEM in the peripheral nerves. Seventy percent of patients with GBS have antecedent infection, including but not limited to campylobacter, CMV, and Epstein-Barr virus (**Figs. 7** and **8**). GBS has several different clinical subtypes, including acute inflammatory demyelinating polyradiculoneuropathy (AIDP), acute motor axonal neuropathy (AMAN), and acute motor sensory axonal neuropathy (AMSAN).

On pathologic examination, AIDP typically shows demyelination of the peripheral nerves, predominantly involving the motor neurons but sometimes also sensory nerves. However, AMAN mainly shows axonal degeneration, selectively involving the motor nerves and showing a typical electrophysiologic pattern of axonal injury. Other clinical presentations of AMAN are similar to those of AIDP. Sensory nerves are usually not affected. AMSAN is a severe form of AMAN that involves axons of motor and sensory nerves.

GBS is the most common cause of acute flaccid paralysis. Acute motor weakness of limbs presents symmetrically and progresses from lower to upper limbs. Swallowing and respiratory muscle

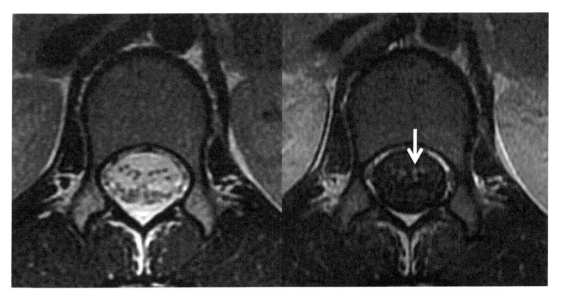

Fig. 7. Guillain-Barré syndrome in an 11-year-old girl with progressive motor weakness 1 week after a cat scratch, which may be the source of the antecedent infection. The ventral roots are predominantly enhanced (*arrow*).

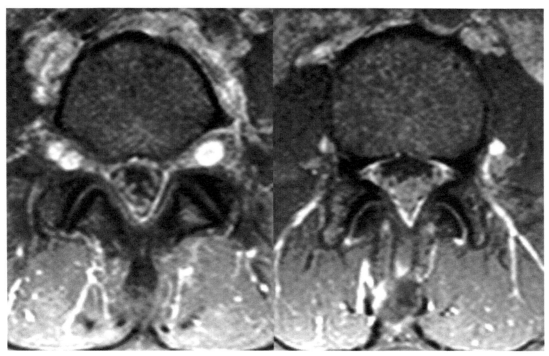

Fig. 8. Guillain-Barré syndrome in a 31-year-old woman with pain in the bilateral thighs and hips. The dorsal and ventral roots are enhanced simultaneously. IgM for CMV was increased in this patient. CMV radiculitis could not be completely excluded based only on imaging studies.

paralyses can develop in severe cases. Cranial and autonomic nerves can also be involved.[24]

GBS is mainly diagnosed based on CSF analysis, electrophysiologic tests, and serum antibodies. Albuminocytologic dissociation is a characteristic finding in a CSF test. Nerve conduction studies and needle electromyography can distinguish demyelination from axonal injury. The presence of serum antiganglioside antibodies is a key factor in making a diagnosis of AMAN and AMSAN.

MR imaging can detect certain characteristic features of GBS, although MR imaging can be nonspecific. Enhancement of the nerve roots is a typical finding. Ventral roots are prone to involvement, although dorsal roots can also show enhancement. Swelling of the nerve roots is usually mild.[25–27]

Enhancement of the nerve roots, however, is observed in many other diseases, such as chronic inflammatory demyelinating polyneuropathy, sarcoidosis, meningitis, meningeal dissemination, lymphoma, spinal cord infarction, ADEM, Krabbe disease, paraneoplastic syndrome, and familial amyloid polyneuropathy.[26] Predominant involvement of the ventral roots is a characteristic and useful finding for reaching a differential diagnosis, although the ventral and dorsal roots are sometimes simultaneously involved in GBS. Finally,

GBS rarely presents with demyelinating foci of the central nervous system, such as the cerebral white matter and the optic nerves.[28]

Acute Transverse Myelitis

ATM is not a specific disease but a syndrome presenting with rapidly progressing paraplegia, sensory disturbance, and bowel or bladder dysfunction, without a compressive cord lesion (**Fig. 9**).[29,30] ATM is divided into idiopathic and secondary types. Idiopathic ATM usually occurs as a postinfectious complication induced by autoimmune processes. This pathogenesis of ATM is quite similar to that of ADEM. The time from onset to completion of symptoms ranges from 4 hours to 3 weeks. Cases with a shorter time course often represent vascular diseases, whereas cases with a longer time course may be neoplastic or degenerative in cause.

Secondary ATM is caused by various factors, such as viral infections, collagen vascular disease, and postvaccination syndrome. Viral myelitis is included in secondary ATM. Some reports also include multiple sclerosis and neuromyelitis optica as causes of ATM. Although these diseases must be separated from ATM, differentiation can be difficult at the first visit.[31]

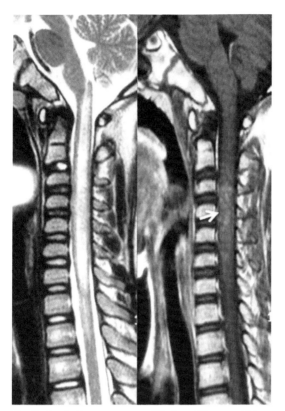

Fig. 9. Acute transverse myelitis in a 10-year-old boy with pain in the bilateral shoulders and upper limbs after influenza infection 1 month ago. The T2-weighted image shows a long segmental lesion extending from the medulla oblongata to C7. A contrast-enhanced T1-weighted image shows punctate enhancing foci (*arrow*).

On imaging, ATM can show intramedullary signal changes extending longitudinally over two spinal segments and two-thirds of the area of the spinal cord. Swelling of the spinal cord is a common feature, although this tends to be milder than with spinal cord tumors. One-third of cases have multiple discontinuous lesions. Enhancement is noted to various extents.[32] Differentiation from ADEM is based on the existence of brain lesions.

CHRONIC MYELITIS
Human T-Lymphotropic Virus Type 1–Associated Myelopathy

HAM is the typical chronic myelopathy that is associated with viral infection. In endemic areas of HTLV-1, HAM is the most common viral myelopathy (**Fig. 10**).[33] HAM affects less than 2% of HTLV-1 carriers. Although the detailed pathogenesis of HAM is not yet clear, activation of lymphocytes caused by HTLV-1 infection and immunity against infected lymphocytes are considered to

be related to injury to the spinal cord.[34] A high provirus load is an important risk factor. In addition, gene polymorphisms in the interleukin-10 promoter and in interleukin-28B are related to HAM. The onset is usually insidious but may be sudden.

The main neurologic manifestations are chronic spastic paraparesis that usually progresses slowly, hyperreflexia, ankle clonus, extensor plantar responses, and lumbar pain. The presence of HTLV-1 antibodies or antigens in blood and CSF is required for diagnosis. In addition, the HTLV-1 proviral load in the central nervous system has been proposed as a new parameter.

Demyelination, necrosis, and cellular infiltration into the perivascular space and subarachnoid space are seen mainly in the lateral and dorsal columns. Cellular infiltration and gliosis of the gray matter are also observed. The thoracic cord is relatively vulnerable to HAM.

On MR imaging, swelling can be detected during the early phase.[35] In the chronic phase, typical imaging findings are limited to cord atrophy.[36,37] In cases with signal abnormalities, the lateral column is relatively easily observed as being involved. On brain MR imaging, cerebral white matter lesions may be observed.[36]

Involvement of the lateral columns can be nonspecific because this is also seen in amyotrophic lateral sclerosis, subacute combined degeneration, cerebrotendinous xanthomatosis, adrenoleukomyelopathy, and wallerian degeneration caused by motor nerve damage. HTLV-1–associated radiculopathy without myelopathy has also been reported.

Human Immunodeficiency Virus–Associated Myelopathy

Vacuolar myelopathy is the most common myelopathy associated with HIV. This type of myelopathy predominantly affects patients with low numbers of CD4-positive cells (**Fig. 11**). Around 20% to 55% of patients have this myelopathy on pathologic examination, although only 5% to 10% are symptomatic.[38] HIV may directly affect the spinal cord, but the pathogenesis of vacuolar myelopathy remains unclear.

Clinical symptoms include slowly progressive spastic paraparesis, sensory ataxia, and neurogenic bladder. No specific markers for vacuolar myelopathy exist. Other types of pathogenesis must be excluded, such as toxoplasmosis, CMV, VZV, cryptococcus, and tuberculosis. The dorsal and lateral columns of the thoracic cord are particularly affected in vacuolar myelopathy.

On MR imaging, atrophy and signal changes can be detected. Spinal cord signal abnormalities mainly affect the white matter. However, the

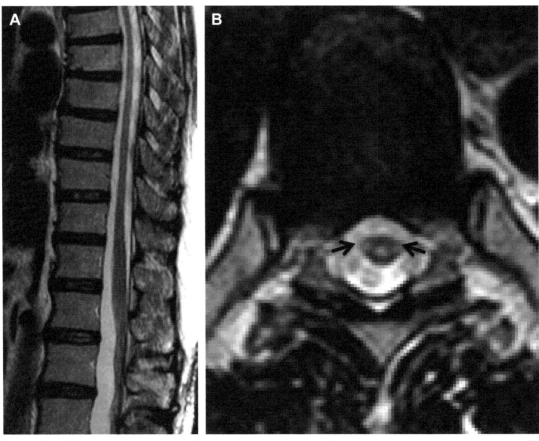

Fig. 10. (A) HTLV-1–associated myelopathy in a 45-year-old man with spastic paraparesis for 10 years. The T2-weighted image shows spinal cord atrophy, especially in the thoracic cord. Abnormal signals are not seen on axial images. (B) Another case of a 50-year-old man with spastic quadriparesia and dysuria. Atrophic thoracic cord with hyperintensity of both lateral columns (arrows) and the central portion is revealed.

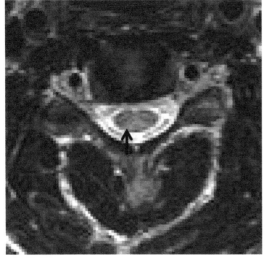

Fig. 11. HIV-associated vacuolar myelopathy in a 29-year-old man with slowly progressive paraparesis and sensory disturbance. The dorsal column shows hyperintensity on the T2-weighted image (arrow).

abnormalities are often diffuse without a specific distribution pattern.[38–40] In some cases, vacuolar myelopathy with signal change in the dorsal column can appear very similar to subacute combined degeneration.[41] In fact, vitamin B_{12} deficiency occurs in 13% to 50% of HIV-infected patients, and thus, the differentiation of the two conditions can be a clinical challenge when patients with HIV present with symmetric signal changes in the dorsal columns. Other differential diagnoses include folic acid deficiency, copper deficiency, wallerian degeneration caused by sensory nerve damage, and intrathecal chemotherapy.

SUMMARY

Familiarity with clinical, pathologic, and imaging findings of viral myelopathy and radiculopathy is useful for correct diagnosis. The time course and anatomic distribution are particularly important for determining the differential diagnosis.

REFERENCES

1. Irani DN. Aseptic meningitis and viral myelitis. Neurol Clin 2008;26:635–55, vii–viii.
2. Leite C, Barbosa A Jr, Lucato LT. Viral diseases of the central nervous system. Top Magn Reson Imaging 2005;16:189–212.
3. Lo CP, Chen CY. Neuroimaging of viral infections in infants and young children. Neuroimaging Clin N Am 2008;18:119–32, viii.
4. Mihai C, Jubelt B. Infectious myelitis. Curr Neurol Neurosci Rep 2012;12:633–41.
5. Grayev AM, Kissane J, Kanekar S. Imaging approach to the cord T2 hyperintensity (myelopathy). Radiol Clin North Am 2014;52:427–46.
6. Devinsky O, Cho ES, Petito CK, et al. Herpes zoster myelitis. Brain 1991;114(Pt 3):1181–96.
7. Friedman DP. Herpes zoster myelitis: MR appearance. AJNR Am J Neuroradiol 1992;13:1404–6.
8. Gilden DH, Beinlich BR, Rubinstien EM, et al. Varicella-zoster virus myelitis: an expanding spectrum. Neurology 1994;44:1818–23.
9. Zijdewind JM, Dijkmans AC, Purmer IM, et al. An aggressive case of PCR negative varicella zoster virus induced transverse myelitis. Neurol Sci 2014;35:961–3.
10. Kornreich L, Dagan O, Grunebaum M. MRI in acute poliomyelitis. Neuroradiology 1996;38:371–2.
11. Malzberg MS, Rogg JM, Tate CA, et al. Poliomyelitis: hyperintensity of the anterior horn cells on MR images of the spinal cord. AJR Am J Roentgenol 1993;161:863–5.
12. Dalakas M, Illa I. Post-polio syndrome: concepts in clinical diagnosis, pathogenesis, and etiology. Adv Neurol 1991;56:495–511.
13. Grafman J, Clark K, Richardson D, et al. Neuropsychology of post-polio syndrome. Ann N Y Acad Sci 1995;753:103–10.
14. Sorenson EJ, Daube JR, Windebank AJ. A 15-year follow-up of neuromuscular function in patients with prior poliomyelitis. Neurology 2005;64:1070–2.
15. Chen CY, Chang YC, Huang CC, et al. Acute flaccid paralysis in infants and young children with enterovirus 71 infection: MR imaging findings and clinical correlates. AJNR Am J Neuroradiol 2001;22:200–5.
16. Jang S, Suh SI, Ha SM, et al. Enterovirus 71-related encephalomyelitis: usual and unusual magnetic resonance imaging findings. Neuroradiology 2012;54:239–45.
17. Shen WC, Chiu HH, Chow KC, et al. MR imaging findings of enteroviral encephaloymelitis: an outbreak in Taiwan. AJNR Am J Neuroradiol 1999;20:1889–95.
18. Solomon T, Kneen R, Dung NM, et al. Poliomyelitis-like illness due to Japanese encephalitis virus. Lancet 1998;351:1094–7.
19. Banwell B, Kennedy J, Sadovnick D, et al. Incidence of acquired demyelination of the CNS in Canadian children. Neurology 2009;72:232–9.
20. Leake JA, Albani S, Kao AS, et al. Acute disseminated encephalomyelitis in childhood: epidemiologic, clinical and laboratory features. Pediatr Infect Dis J 2004;23:756–64.
21. Murthy SN, Faden HS, Cohen ME, et al. Acute disseminated encephalomyelitis in children. Pediatrics 2002;110:e21.
22. Honkaniemi J, Dastidar P, Kahara V, et al. Delayed MR imaging changes in acute disseminated encephalomyelitis. AJNR Am J Neuroradiol 2001;22:1117–24.
23. Kinoshita A, Hayashi M, Miyamoto K, et al. Inflammatory demyelinating polyradiculitis in a patient with acute disseminated encephalomyelitis (ADEM). J Neurol Neurosurg Psychiatry 1996;60:87–90.
24. Alshekhlee A, Hussain Z, Sultan B, et al. Guillain-Barre syndrome: incidence and mortality rates in US hospitals. Neurology 2008;70:1608–13.
25. Georgy BA, Chong B, Chamberlain M, et al. MR of the spine in Guillain-Barre syndrome. AJNR Am J Neuroradiol 1994;15:300–1.
26. Georgy BA, Snow RD, Hesselink JR. MR imaging of spinal nerve roots: techniques, enhancement patterns, and imaging findings. AJR Am J Roentgenol 1996;166:173–9.
27. Perry JR, Fung A, Poon P, et al. Magnetic resonance imaging of nerve root inflammation in the Guillain-Barre syndrome. Neuroradiology 1994;36:139–40.
28. An JY, Yoon B, Kim JS, et al. Guillain-Barre syndrome with optic neuritis and a focal lesion in the central white matter following Epstein-Barr virus infection. Intern Med 2008;47:1539–42.
29. Bhargava P, Elble RJ. Clinical reasoning: an unusual cause of transverse myelitis? Neurology 2014;82:e46–50.
30. Scott TF, Frohman EM, De Seze J, et al. Evidence-based guideline: clinical evaluation and treatment of transverse myelitis: report of the therapeutics and technology assessment subcommittee of the American Academy of Neurology. Neurology 2011;77:2128–34.
31. Bourre B, Zephir H, Ongagna JC, et al. Long-term follow-up of acute partial transverse myelitis. Arch Neurol 2012;69:357–62.
32. Goh C, Desmond PM, Phal PM. MRI in transverse myelitis. J Magn Reson Imaging 2014;40(6):1267–79.
33. Kamei S, Takasu T. Nationwide survey of the annual prevalence of viral and other neurological infections in Japanese inpatients. Intern Med 2000;39:894–900.
34. Araujo AQ, Silva MT. The HTLV-1 neurological complex. Lancet Neurol 2006;5:1068–76.
35. Shakudo M, Inoue Y, Tsutada T. HTLV-1-associated myelopathy: acute progression and atypical MR findings. AJNR Am J Neuroradiol 1999;20:1417–21.

36. Kira J, Fujihara K, Itoyama Y, et al. Leukoencephal-opathy in HTLV-1-associated myelopathy/tropical spastic paraparesis: MRI analysis and a two year follow-up study after corticosteroid therapy. J Neurol Sci 1991;106:41–9.

37. Melo A, Moura L, Rios S, et al. Magnetic resonance imaging in HTLV-1 associated myelopathy. Arq Neuropsiquiatr 1993;51:329–32.

38. McArthur JC, Brew BJ, Nath A. Neurological complications of HIV infection. Lancet Neurol 2005;4:543–55.

39. Anneken K, Fischera M, Evers S, et al. Recurrent vacuolar myelopathy in HIV infection. J Infect 2006;52:e181–3.

40. Santosh CG, Bell JE, Best JJ. Spinal tract pathology in AIDS: postmortem MRI correlation with neuropathology. Neuroradiology 1995;37:134–8.

41. Sartoretti-Schefer S, Blattler T, Wichmann W. Spinal MRI in vacuolar myelopathy, and correlation with histopathological findings. Neuroradiology 1997;39:865–9.

Parasitic and Rare Spinal Infections

Lázaro Luís Faria do Amaral, MD[a,b,*], Renato Hoffmann Nunes, MD[a,c],
Antonio Jose da Rocha, MD, PhD[a,c]

KEYWORDS

- Spine • Parasitic • Infection • Tropical disorders • MR imaging • Central nervous system

KEY POINTS

- Despite the reporting of uncommon diseases, often with similar patterns, infectious diseases are usually treatable, and radiologists may play a pivotal role in the appropriate diagnostic workup.
- The most common parasitic disease involving the central nervous system is cysticercosis; however, spinal cord schistosomiasis is also an important diagnosis in endemic regions. Additionally, toxoplasmosis is a common pathogen in immunocompromised patients.
- This article discusses key features of trypanosomiases and echinococcosis. Additionally, several nonparasitic diseases are herein discussed, including syphilis, Baggio-Yoshinari syndrome, paracoccidioidomycosis, and HTLV-1–associated myelopathy.

INTRODUCTION

A large number of agents can produce spinal lesions. Among these, bacteria are the most common agents, although other rarer organisms also can cause spinal injuries. Our current aim is to discuss the imaging features of spinal parasitic diseases and other rare infectious diseases, with an emphasis on spinal cord involvement. Despite the reporting of uncommon diseases, often with similar patterns, infectious diseases are usually treatable, and radiologists may play a pivotal role in the appropriate diagnostic workup by interfacing with clinicians and facilitating direct, appropriate testing for early diagnosis and correct treatment.[1]

Despite the development of modern magnetic resonance (MR) techniques, these approaches are less useful for the detection of spinal cord involvement. Detailed analysis of structural images remains the main source of data for presumed diagnosis; however, diffusion-weighted images and constructive interference with the steady-state technique contribute to diagnosis in some specific cases herein described.

The most common parasitic conditions affecting the anatomic compartments of the spine are herein described. Subsequently, several rare infectious pathogenic agents are discussed individually with respect to their effect on the spine and its contents.

PARASITIC DISEASES

Parasitic diseases are distributed worldwide, with an increased prevalence in areas with poor sanitary conditions and developing countries. Nevertheless, in nonendemic areas, sporadic cases may occur as a consequence of increased international travel and immunocompromising conditions. A variety of parasitic diseases can involve the central nervous system (CNS), with multiple clinical presentations.[2] The most common of these diseases is cysticercosis, although in endemic

Disclosure Statement: All authors report no disclosures.
[a] Division of Neuroradiology, Santa Casa de Misericórdia de São Paulo, Rua Cesário Motta Júnior, 112, Vila Buarque, São Paulo, São Paulo 01221-020, Brazil; [b] Division of Neuroradiology, MEDIMAGEM - Hospital da Beneficência Portuguesa de São Paulo, Rua Luiz Gottschalk, 151, Apartment 111 MS, Vila Mariana, São Paulo, São Paulo 04008-070, Brazil; [c] Division of Neuroradiology, Fleury Medicina e Saúde, Rua Cincinato Braga, 282, Bela Vista, São Paulo, São Paulo 01333-010, Brazil
* Corresponding author. MEDIMAGEM - Hospital da Beneficência Portuguesa de São Paulo, Rua Luiz Gottschalk, 151, Apartment 111 MS, Vila Mariana, São Paulo, São Paulo 04008-070, Brazil.
E-mail address: lazden@terra.com.br

neuroimaging.theclinics.com

regions, schistosomiasis is also a common cause of spinal cord syndrome.[1] Additionally, toxoplasmosis is a frequent CNS pathogen in immunocompromised patients, particularly in patients with acquired immunodeficiency syndrome (AIDS), but it rarely involves the spinal cord.[3]

Trypanosomiases and echinococcosis are also emerging parasitic diseases in some parts of the world. Although the definite diagnosis of a spinal parasitosis is usually confirmed based on histopathology, the clinical suspicion is generally based on a combination of ethnic, clinical, serologic, and neuroimaging features.

Neurocysticercosis

Overview

Cysticercosis is caused by implantation of the cestode *Taenia solium* (pork tapeworm) in humans, which serve as an intermediate host. This disease affects approximately 50 million people worldwide, with a prevalence of 3% to 6% of the population in endemic areas, including Central and South America, Eastern Europe, Africa, and some regions in Asia.[4] Neurocysticercosis (NCC) has become an increasingly important emerging infection in the United States, largely due to the influx of immigrants from endemic regions.[5]

Pathophysiology

Cysticercosis occurs as a result of ingestion of eggs by humans, which serve as incidental intermediate dead-end hosts. Embryos are released in the small intestine, which are subsequently lysed by gastric juices and invade the bowel wall to reach the arterial system. Then, the parasites lodge preferentially in neural and subcutaneous tissues, as well as in the skeletal muscles and ocular globes, where they continue to develop. In the CNS, the oncospheres develop into a secondary larval form called cysticerci over a period of 3 weeks to 2 months.[4] The larval stage of this organism may become disseminated throughout all CNS compartments.

The most common larval form is *Cysticercus cellulosae*, which characteristically has a scolex and causes brain intraparenchymal lesions or, rarely, spinal intramedullary lesions. *Cysticercus racemosae*, which lacks a scolex, usually grows in grapelike clusters of thin-walled cysts and shows a tendency to predominate in the subarachnoid space.[1] However, this terminology does not help with diagnosis from an imaging point of view because these organisms are both forms of the same parasite, commonly coexisting in a single patient.[5]

The macroscopic appearance of cysticerci varies according to their location in the CNS. Cysticerci, in most cases, remain small, approximately 1 cm in diameter, and tend to lodge in the cerebral cortex or the basal ganglia.[5] The Sylvian fissure and basal cisterns are the most common locations of subarachnoid cysticerci, where they may reach 10 cm or more (**Fig. 1**A).[6]

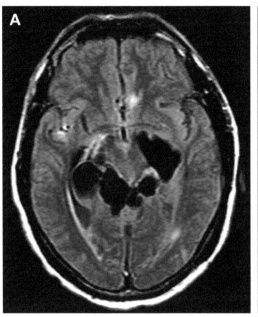 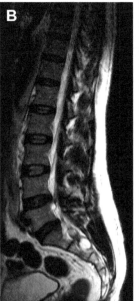 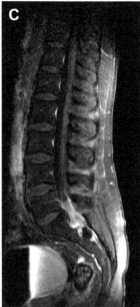

Fig. 1. Disseminated subarachnoid cysticercosis. (*A*) The axial fluid-attenuated inversion recovery (FLAIR) image showed numerous cysts distending and distorting the perimesencephalic and quadrigeminal cisterns. (*B*) The sagittal T2WI and (*C*) fat-sat postcontrast T1WI demonstrated multiple cysts in the spinal subarachnoid space and evidence of acute arachnoiditis.

Clinical manifestations

The clinical presentation of cysticercosis is often nonspecific, depending on the number and location of parasitic organisms and the ensuing inflammatory reaction. Degeneration of the cyst is usually associated with a mass effect and edema, resulting in focal neurologic symptoms; when this process occurs in the brain, seizures typically ensue.[5]

Diagnosis

The proposed diagnostic criteria include epidemiologic factors and the results of physical examination, funduscopy, serologic tests, and imaging.[7] Additionally, imaging plays a main role in confirming and fully characterizing the different forms of NCC.[8]

Imaging

Four stages of development and regression have been described for NCC using both computed tomography (CT) and MR imaging, with histopathologic correlation (**Table 1**). Notably, multiple anatomic sites are simultaneously involved, which is not uncommon in various stages of the disease.[5,9] Severe forms of presentation with seizures or focal neurologic deficits are usually characterized on images by extensive vasogenic edema and contrast enhancement (colloidal or nodular-granular stages) and are represented by an isolated lesion in subcortical areas. Conversely, multifocal parenchymal lesions often do not elicit an inflammatory reaction, and most of the parasites in such cases remain alive. Subarachnoid cysticercosis lesions are often multiple and contain live parasites.

Spinal neurocysticercosis

Extradural lesions are extremely rare, whereas spinal cord involvement is considered very uncommon and is reported in only 1.2% to 5.8% of patients with NCC.[10] Furthermore, the leptomeningeal form occurs 6 to 8 times more often than the intramedullary form.[5]

Presumably, intradural-extramedullary (**Fig. 2**) involvement is a consequence of the downward migration of larvae from the intracranial compartment to the spinal subarachnoid space (see **Fig. 1B, C**), and the cysts may remain mobile in this region (**Fig. 3**). Similar to brain parenchymal lesions, intramedullary cysticercosis (**Fig. 4**) typically arises from the hematogenous dissemination of larva, particularly in the thoracic cord, as a consequence of its vascular supply.[10]

Neurologic manifestations may arise from an inflammatory reaction caused by parasitic metabolites, degenerated larva, the mass effect from intramedullary or extramedullary cysts (see **Figs. 2 and 4**), leptomeningitis (see **Fig. 1C; Fig. 5**), or vascular insufficiency.[5]

MR imaging is the most useful modality to evaluate spinal NCC, as this approach can reveal the intensity of the viable cystic fluid, which (whether in the spinal cord or the subarachnoid space) is usually similar to that of the cerebrospinal fluid (CSF) on both T1-weighted images (WIs) and T2WIs. MR further demonstrates mass effects, variable vesicular enhancement, and adjacent edema as a result of dead larvae. The absence of a CSF flow void is commonly observed adjacent to extramedullary cysts. High-resolution highly T2-weighted sequences, such as the use of constructive interference in steady-state (3-dimensional constructive interference in steady-state [3D-CISS]) techniques, allow for better delineation of the cyst and its scolex, when it is present (see **Figs. 2 and 4C**). Cisternal MR imaging, as in myelography (see **Fig. 3**), enables detection of the cyst, which appears as a hypointense cystic wall surrounded by contrast material.[2,5]

However, the MR imaging features of intramedullary NCC are not specific in the absence of the scolex, and the differential diagnosis includes neoplastic, inflammatory, demyelinating, vascular, and granulomatous lesions. Marked eosinophilia may be useful for differentiation from a spinal arachnoid cyst.[10] Intramedullary NCC also may occur in conjunction with cysticercal meningitis and intracranial lesions, which should be recognized.[5]

Table 1 Stages of neurocysticercosis	
First stage	
Vesicular	Cyst and scolex.
Second stage	
Colloidal	Ring enhancement and edema.
Third stage	
Nodular-granular	Decreased enhancement and edema. Initiation of calcification.
Fourth stage	
Calcified	Calcification on CT or MR imaging.[a]

Abbreviation: CT, computed tomography.

[a] Reactive inflammation in calcified lesions has been observed with recurrent edema and peripheral enhancement, mainly in a quiescent brain lesion.

Data from do Amaral LL, Ferreira RM, da Rocha AJ, et al. Neurocysticercosis: evaluation with advanced magnetic resonance techniques and atypical forms. Top Magn Reson Imaging 2005;16(2):127–44; and Dumas JL, Visy JM, Belin C, et al. Parenchymal neurocysticercosis: follow-up and staging by MRI. Neuroradiology 1997;39(1):12–8.

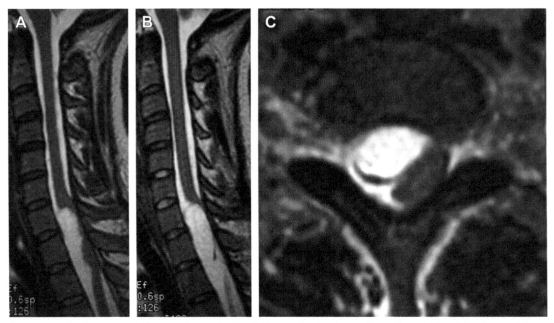

Fig. 2. Intradural-extramedullary cysticercosis. (*A, B*) The sagittal volumetric T2WI and (*C*) axial volumetric T2WI demonstrated a cystic lesion in the intradural compartment displacing the spinal cord.

Schistosomiasis

Overview

Spinal schistosomiasis, the best-known form of neuroschistosomiasis, is a severe, underrecognized form of schistosomiasis that occurs at any time during the parasitic infestation.[11]

Schistosomiasis is one of the most widespread parasitic diseases worldwide and is an important public health problem, particularly in tropical areas. Approximately 200 million people worldwide are afflicted with schistosomiasis, and approximately 20 million develop severe disease, including CNS forms.[12] Neuroschistosomiasis has been increasingly reported not only in endemic areas but also in Western countries, owing to immigration and international travel.[13]

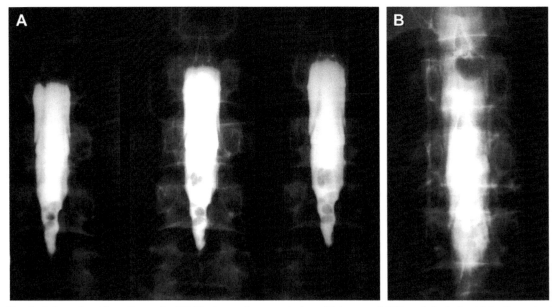

Fig. 3. Subarachnoid cysticercosis. (*A*) Myelography revealed multiple round filling defects (cysts) in the spinal subarachnoid space. (*B*) After the Trendelenburg maneuver, the cysts moved to a higher position, confirming their mobility.

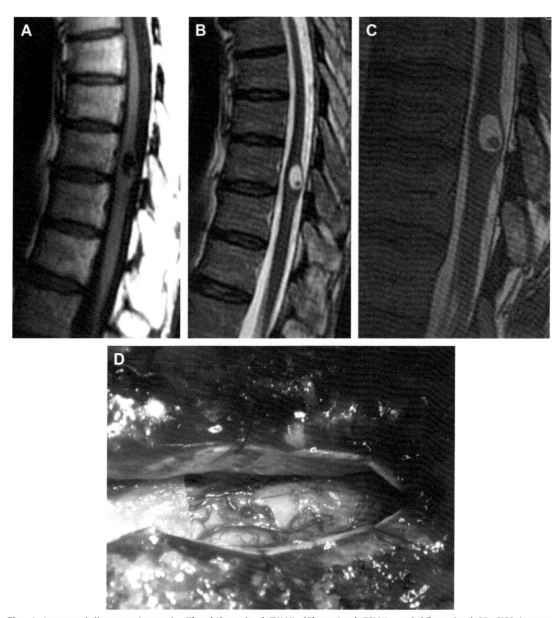

Fig. 4. Intramedullary cysticercosis. The (*A*) sagittal T1WI, (*B*) sagittal T2WI, and (*C*) sagittal 3D-CISS images demonstrated an intramedullary cystic lesion with thick, identifiable cyst walls and an eccentric scolex. (*D*) Intraoperative findings. (*Courtesy of* F. Gonçalves, MD, Brasília-DF, Brazil.)

Pathophysiology

Almost all reported cases of neuroschistosomiasis are caused by infection with *Schistosoma mansoni*, consequent to a parasite configuration that makes retrograde migration from the abdominal veins to Batson plexus difficult. Whereas *Schistosoma haematobium* primarily affects the urinary tract, *Schistosoma japonicum* has an increased likelihood of extending to the brain parenchyma.

Since the first description of this disease in the 1930s, approximately 800 cases have been reported, most of them due to *S mansoni*.[14]

Neurologic symptoms may result from the deposition of eggs surrounded by granulomatous reactions in circumscribed areas of the brain or spinal cord, although the simultaneous occurrence of cerebral and spinal schistosomiasis is extremely rare.[15]

Clinical manifestations

In endemic areas, spinal schistosomiasis is more common in children, adolescents, and young adults; however, with the exception of hepatomegaly (present in 25% of the patients), these

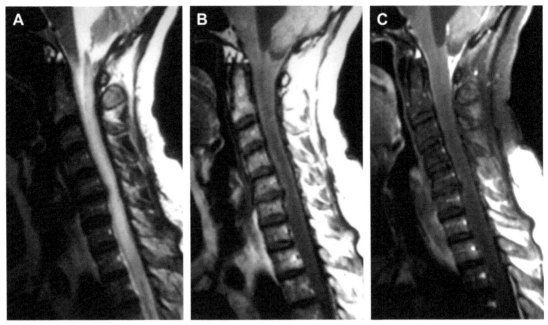

Fig. 5. Extensive meningitis due to NCC. (*A*) The sagittal T2WI displayed cervical spinal cord edema. (*B*) The sagittal pregadolinium T1WI and (*C*) postgadolinium image demonstrated leptomeningeal and pachymeningeal enhancement and thickening, leading to spinal cord compression.

patients rarely show any other symptoms. The disease usually presents acutely or subacutely as conus medullary syndrome and is often associated with the involvement of cauda equina roots.[14]

Clinically, spinal cord schistosomiasis may be classified into 3 classic forms (summarized in **Table 2**); however, the disease can progress from one form to another.[14] The medullary form is generally associated with a rapid course and severe weakness. By contrast, in conus-cauda equina syndrome, the symptoms develop more slowly, the distribution of the sensorimotor alterations is predominantly asymmetric, and the muscle weakness is less severe.[14]

Diagnosis
Laminectomy with biopsy of the nervous tissue is the only method that provides a definite diagnosis of spinal schistosomiasis; however, to prevent sequelae, this procedure should be avoided. Blood eosinophilia, antibody levels, and the presence of parasite ova in the urine and/or stool may not be detectable at disease onset.[11] CSF examination usually reveals nonspecific abnormalities that may be found in other parasite infections, including eosinophils.[14] The detection of antibodies to schistosomes in the CSF by enzyme-linked immunosorbent assay (ELISA) is specific for the diagnosis of *S mansoni*, although further validation of this technique has been recommended.[11,14]

Although its clinical picture is nonspecific, spinal schistosomiasis should be strongly considered in young patients presenting with acute paraplegia, myeloradicular pain syndrome, or cauda equina syndrome with a positive epidemiologic origin. The clinical diagnosis becomes less likely when higher segments are affected or when the symptoms progress more slowly. A rapid and pronounced improvement after treatment lends further support to diagnosis.[14] The differential diagnosis of spinal schistosomiasis should include ependymoma, spinal cord astrocytoma, metastatic tumors, and venous congestion in a spinal dural arteriovenous fistula.[11]

Imaging
Although the alterations observed in cases of spinal schistosomiasis are usually nonspecific, MR imaging greatly contributes to the diagnosis, easily demonstrating the abnormalities in the spinal cord and helping to rule out the differential diagnosis. Although clinical forms usually coexist (see **Table 2**), the most common imaging findings are described in the medullary form and the conus syndrome (see **Fig. 6**), which is characterized by a patchy pattern hyperintensity on T2WIs, enlargement of the spinal cord, and a remarkable heterogeneous contrast enhancement on T1WIs, particularly in the lower cord and conus medullaris.[2,11,14,16,17] This interesting multinodular enhancing pattern is associated with multiple schistosome eggs and granulomas in

Table 2
Spinal schistosomiasis forms

Clinical Forms	Clinical Manifestations	Imaging
Medullary: predominantly spinal cord involvement.	Rapid course, severe weakness, and a symmetric distribution of the sensorimotor abnormalities. May present with high eosinophil levels in the CSF.	T2 hyperintensity and enlargement of the spinal cord associated with mild and heterogeneous enhancement.
Conus-cauda equine syndrome: mainly conus medullaris or cauda equina involvement (Fig. 6).	Symptoms develop more slowly, muscle weakness is less severe, and the distribution of the sensorimotor alterations is predominantly asymmetric. Usually presents with high eosinophil levels in the CSF.	Enlargement and heterogeneous gadolinium enhancement of the conus medullaris. Thickening of the cauda equina.
Myeloradicular: predominantly spinal cord and nerve root involvement (Fig. 7).	This is the most common presentation and represents an intermediate form of presentation. Often begins with lumbalgia and pain in the lower limbs (radiculopathy) followed by muscular weakness and sensory disturbances in the lower limbs. Usually presents with high eosinophil levels in the CSF.	Thickening of the spinal nerve roots and leptomeningeal enhancement. Epidural venous plexus congestion might also be identified.

Abbreviation: CSF, cerebrospinal fluid.

Data from Ferrari TC, Moreira PR. Neuroschistosomiasis: clinical symptoms and pathogenesis. Lancet Neurol 2011;10(9):853–64.

the spinal cord, peripheral contrast enhancement with eggs, and granulomas in the leptomeninges.[16] In addition, this appearance may mimic a cord neoplasm.[1]

Occasionally, MR imaging also may display an intramedullary arborized appearance, which is highly suggestive of this disease in individuals from endemic schistosomiasis regions.[8,17] In cases with a longer evolution, medullary atrophy can be observed (see Fig. 6D).[8] In the other clinical forms (myeloradicular and cauda equine), MR imaging demonstrates thickening of the spinal roots (especially the cauda equina roots) and a linear radicular contrast enhancement, representing eggs and granulomas on the surface of nerve roots (see Fig. 7).[11,14,16]

Rare forms

The granulomatous form of schistosomiasis results from an intense granulomatous inflammatory reaction around the eggs in association with gliosis and fibrosis. This reaction leads to the formation of focal expanding intra-axial or extra-axial lesions, which demonstrate a pattern of *intense* epidural enhancement adjacent to areas of medullary involvement.[8,18] Extradural compromising (bilharzioma) is considered rare.[19]

Other even rarer forms, which may be revealed by imaging, include acute transverse myelitis (which may be hemorrhagic and necrotizing) and an acute, anterior spinal artery syndrome.[1]

Echinococcosis (Hydatid Disease)

Overview

Hydatid disease (echinococcosis) is a parasitosis caused by the larval stage of *Echinococcus*. Several carnivores and canines are definitive hosts for these parasites and can be found near homes in forest areas or the countryside. Humans are secondarily infected via the ingestion of food or water contaminated by eggs of the parasite. The 2 most frequent clinical forms are cystic echinococcosis, caused by *Echinococcus granulosus*, and, less frequently, alveolar echinococcosis, caused by *Echinococcus multilocularis*.[20]

Hydatid disease remains a health problem in endemic areas of countries in which veterinary control is precarious, mostly in the temperate zones.[20]

This disease is diagnosed by serologic and imaging tests. The most frequently involved organ

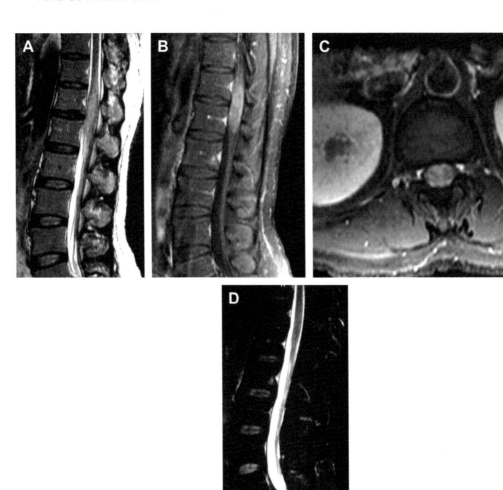

Fig. 6. Neuroschistosomiasis (conus-cauda equine syndrome). The (*A*) sagittal T2WI, and (*B*) sagittal and (*C*) axial fat suppressed (fat-sat) postcontrast T1WI revealed expansion of the conus medullaris associated with spinal cord edema in the affected area associated with heterogeneous enhancement in the areas of medullary involvement. (*D*) The follow-up image after treatment revealed a reduction in the lesion's size.

is the liver, and CNS involvement is rare (1% to 2% of all cases), even in endemic areas.[8,20,21]

Spinal echinococcosis: overview

Spinal involvement in echinococcosis is rare, although the thoracic segment of the spine is the most frequently affected region (50% of cases), followed by the lumbar (20%), sacral (20%), and cervical (10%) segments.[21]

Spinal echinococcosis: clinical and imaging manifestations

The imaging and clinical presentation of spinal echinococcosis depends on the primarily infected anatomic structures.[21] This disease usually manifests as isointense cystic lesions without significant peripheral edema.[22] The fibrous capsule is characteristically hypointense on T2WIs and may display discrete peripheral enhancement in the presence of active inflammation (**Fig. 8**).[23]

Although intramedullar echinococcosis is rare, intradural-extramedullary cysts are more common. These cysts usually grow eccentrically and follow the line of least resistance along the dural sack. Compared with extradural echinococcosis, they are more frequently limited to a single cyst and appear to present at a younger age.[21]

Spinal echinococcosis: differential diagnosis

Intradural-extramedullar or intramedullar cysticerci may mimic echinococcosis.[24] In addition, and even

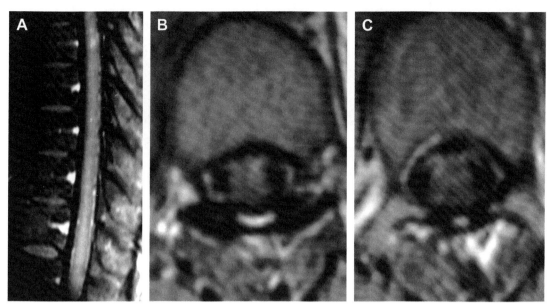

Fig. 7. Neuroschistosomiasis (myeloradicular syndrome). The (A) sagittal and (B, C) axial fat-sat postcontrast T1WI demonstrated leptomeningeal enhancement along the spinal cord surface and thickening of the cauda equina roots.

more rarely, cestode infections also may mimic spinal alveolar echinococcosis (*E multilocularis*) and spinal sparganosis (*Spirometra* sp). Spinal arachnoid cysts and spinal aneurysmal bone cysts also are potential differential diagnoses; however, marked eosinophilia should be useful in confirming a suspicion of parasitic disease.[21]

Toxoplasmosis

Overview
The protozoan *Toxoplasma gondii* is a significant zoonotic pathogen with a global distribution.[25] This obligate intracellular parasite can cross all biological barriers and finally invades the host CNS. The course of toxoplasmosis is well described for maternal primary infection during pregnancy, which can lead to various congenital defects and even abortion, and infection or reactivation of a preexisting infection in immunocompromised individuals, often causing encephalitis.[25,26]

Neurotoxoplasmosis is diagnosed on clinical, serologic, CSF, or imaging investigations. The highest sensitivity can be achieved by the application of polymerase chain reaction methods in the serum or CSF, whereas ELISA or immunoblotting of the CSF demonstrate better specificity.[2,8]

Spinal toxoplasmosis: overview
Although few reports have been published describing spinal toxoplasmosis in humans, adult-acquired toxoplasmosis also can affect the spinal cord. This spinal cord pathology clinically manifests predominantly in severely immunocompromised patients, especially due to CD4 T-cell immune deficits associated with AIDS or T-cell leukemia/lymphoma.[3,27]

Spinal toxoplasmosis: clinical manifestations
Depending on the parasite location (with respect to different segments of the spinal cord), the symptomatology is characterized by motor and sensory loss, urinary sphincter abnormalities, and pain.[26]

Spinal toxoplasmosis: imaging
In patients with AIDS, toxoplasmosis spinal lesions usually present as enhancing intramedullary lesions with an extensive mass effect and associated edema. Frequently, the presence of coexisting cerebral toxoplasma lesions assists in diagnosing the spinal disease (**Figs. 9–11**).[1]

Chagas Disease (American Trypanosomiasis)

Overview
American trypanosomiasis, also known as Chagas disease, occurs primarily in Latin America; however, there have been some reports in other Western countries.[8,28] This disease is caused by *Trypanosoma cruzi*, which is transmitted to humans by blood-sucking insects (Triatominae).[8] Transmission through blood transfusion also has been reported in nonendemic countries without specific tests to detect the intermediate form of disease in asymptomatic donors.[29]

Clinical manifestations
In the acute stages, approximately 35% of patients present nonspecific symptoms, such as

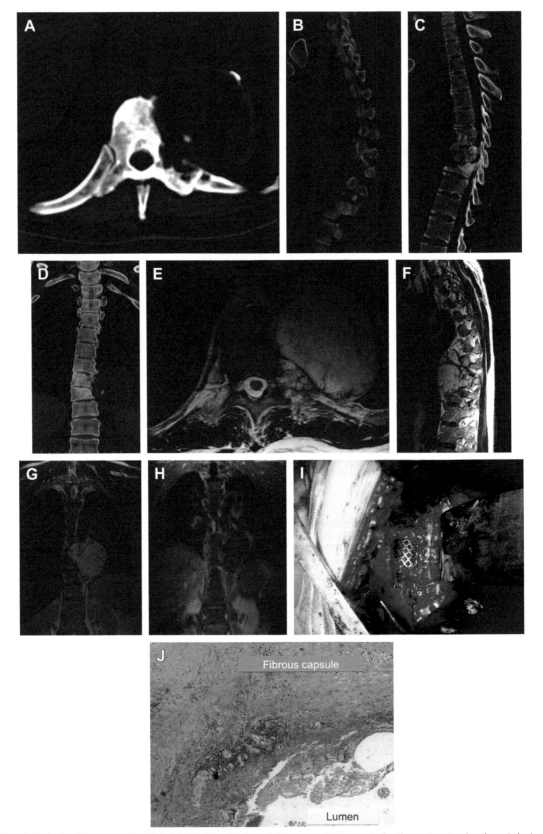

Fig. 8. Spinal echinococcosis. (*A*) Axial, (*B*, *C*) sagittal, and (*D*) coronal CT revealed a thoracic extradural cystic lesion with paravertebral extension and bone erosion. The (*E*) axial, (*F*) sagittal, (*G*) coronal T2WI, and (*H*) coronal fat-sat postcontrast T1WI showed epidural extension and a multicystic appearance (daughter cysts), considered highly suggestive of this disease. (*I*) Extradural cysts were demonstrated in the intraoperative analysis. (*J*) Hematoxylin and eosin staining. A high-magnification micrograph of the cyst wall revealed laminations consistent with those observed in an *Echinococcus* infection (original magnification 100×). (*Courtesy of* A. Abreu, MD, Porto Alegre-RS, Brazil.)

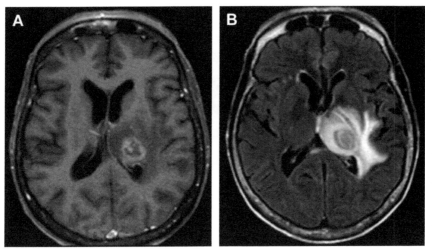

Fig. 9. Neurotoxoplasmosis. The (A) axial fat-sat postcontrast T1WI and (B) axial FLAIR image displayed a left centrencephalic expansive lesion associated with peripheric vasogenic edema and an incomplete annular enhanced area in a patient infected with human immunodeficiency virus (HIV). Typical findings on brain imaging in neurotoxoplasmosis include single or multiple nodular or ring-enhancing lesions with a mass effect and edema and a peripheral target sign. These lesions are characterized by 3 zones: a central zone, an intermediate zone, and a peripheral zone. On T2WI, the lesions may show an eccentric target sign with central hyperintensity due to necrosis, a hypointense rim due to inflammation, and peripheral hyperintensity due to edema.

fever, malaise, headache, lymphadenopathy, and hepatosplenomegaly. The acute phase of disease is usually associated with myocarditis, and clinical signs of CNS involvement rarely occur. Instead, CNS involvement manifests as acute meningitis, which is a hallmark of the disease, or (rarely) as multifocal, nodular encephalitis due to reactivation.[30] Isolated cases with CNS involvement also may present with dementia, confusion, or sensory or motor deficits.[31]

CNS involvement may be a late presentation of the acute phase or caused by reactivation. In the past 2 decades, AIDS has significantly changed the natural course of a variety of infectious diseases, including Chagas disease. Indeed, Chagas meningoencephalitis may manifest as the first presentation of AIDS.[2,31]

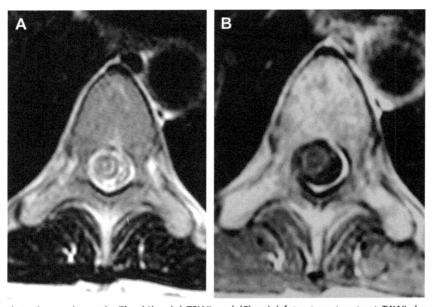

Fig. 10. Spinal cord toxoplasmosis. The (A) axial T2WI and (B) axial fat-sat postcontrast T1WI demonstrated a thoracic intramedullary lesion with peripheral enhancement and T2 hypointensity in an HIV-infected patient with brain toxoplasmosis.

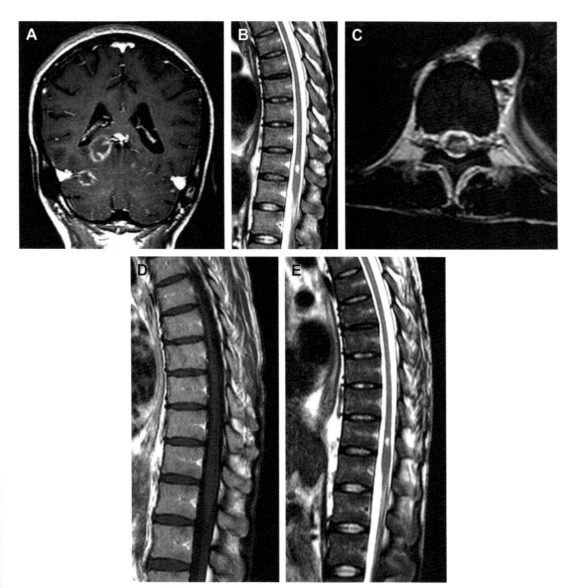

Fig. 11. Neurotoxoplasmosis. (*A*) The coronal T1 fat-sat postcontrast T1WI revealed typical peripheral enhancing supratentorial and infratentorial brain lesions in an HIV-infected patient. (*B*) Sagittal and (*C*) axial T2WIs demonstrated a conus medullary predominantly hyperintense lesion. (*D*) The sagittal fat-sat postcontrast T1WI showed subtle gadolinium enhancement. (*E*) At the 1-month follow-up evaluation after treatment, the sagittal T2WI demonstrated only a sequellary lesion. (*Courtesy of* J.R. Ferraz, MD, Sao Jose do Rio Preto-SP, Brazil.)

Diagnosis

American trypanosomiasis is diagnosed by clinical, serologic, CSF, and imaging findings. Chagas disease is confirmed by serologic and CSF tests for *T cruzi* and histologic examinations. In cases of Chagas meningoencephalitis, appropriate CSF abnormalities can be found.[2]

Imaging

In imaging studies, Chagas meningoencephalitis usually manifests as multiple expanding hyperintense lesions on T2WIs, with nodular or annular enhancement that may occur in the brain parenchyma (corpus callosum, periventricular white matter, or subcortical regions). More rarely, meningoencephalitis also may involve the spinal cord, demonstrating an extensive edema and mass effect (**Fig. 12**).[2,30,32]

Other Rare Parasitic Diseases

Malaria, amebiasis, toxocariasis, and African trypanosomiases are all extremely rare parasitic diseases, and their main characteristics are summarized in **Table 3**.

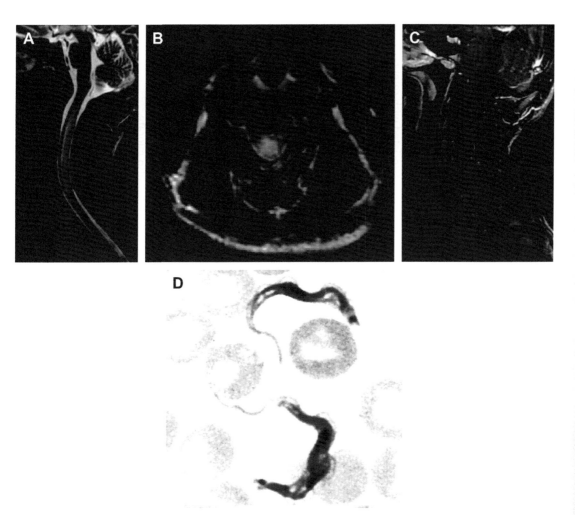

Fig. 12. Spinal cord American trypanosomiasis. (*A*) The sagittal short T1 inversion recovery (STIR) and (*B*) axial T2WI showed a longitudinally extensive cervical spinal cord lesion surrounded by vasogenic edema. (*C*) The sagittal fat-sat postcontrast T1WI revealed subtle posterior enhancement. The imaging findings were not specific but suggested an inflammatory process. (*D*) *Trypanosoma cruzi* in Giemsa stain (original magnification 400×). (*Courtesy of* L.T. Lucato, MD, Sao Paulo-SP, Brazil.)

OTHER AGENTS
Baggio-Yoshinari Syndrome (Lyme Simile)

Overview
In contrast to the Northern Hemisphere's Lyme disease caused by spirochetes belonging to the *Borrelia burgdorferi sensu lato* complex, Baggio-Yoshinari syndrome was first described in Brazil. This disease is transmitted by ticks of the genera *Amblyomma* and/or *Rhipicephalus*, and is caused by spirochetes with an atypical morphology and latent behavior. This infection can lead to systemic and relapsing complications, including immunologic disorders, throughout a prolonged clinical evolution.

Clinical manifestations and imaging
This disease manifests similarly to Lyme disease, specifically in the acute phase, by a characteristic migratory erythema that may emerge associated with symptoms compatible with influenza.[33] After invasion of the cerebral or spinal meninges, neurologic infection is established, which is characterized by the triad of lymphomonocytary meningitis, cranial neuritis, and peripheral radiculopathy, as well as (less commonly) encephalomyelitis.[34,35]

The distinctive clinical aspects of Baggio-Yoshinari syndrome are the high frequency of relapse, especially when patients are not diagnosed and treated early in the acute phase and show neurologic involvement.[34,35]

On MR imaging, this syndrome may present a picture highly similar to Lyme disease (**Fig. 13**). Additional intracranial findings, such as multifocal hyperintense lesions on T2WIs with or without contrast enhancement on T1WIs, simulating demyelinating lesions and different types of cranial nerve

Table 3
Other rare spinal parasitic diseases

Disease	Agent	Distribution	Spinal Cord Manifestations	Imaging
Malariasis	*Plasmodium* sp	Endemic areas in tropical countries	Rarely involves the spine. Acute disseminated encephalomyelitislike symptoms are the most common spinal presentation.	Spinal cord malariasis: longitudinal extensive spinal cord lesion with mild or no enhancement. May present nerve root enhancement. May be associated with cerebral malariasis (cerebral edema, cortical and subcortical ischemic lesions, and multiple petechial hemorrhages).[53]
African trypanosomiasis (sleeping sickness)	*Trypanosoma brucei*	Central and Western Africa	Meningoencephalitis is the most dominant clinical picture. Rarely, myelopathy is the main clinical picture.	Meningeal enhancement and thickening associated with diffuse white matter and basal ganglia lesions.[54]
Neurotoxocariasis	*Toxocara* sp	Worldwide	Myelitis, meningoradiculitis, and arachnoiditis associated with eosinophilic meningitis. May also present with optic neuritis.	Imaging may reveal longitudinal extensive myelopathy or even single or multiple hyperintense lesions on T2WIs with focal nodular enhancement on the posterior or posterolateral segments of the spinal cord that may also migrate.[55,56]
Amebiasis	Free-living amebae (*Entamoeba histolytica; Naegleria fowleri; Acanthamoeba; Balamuthia mandrillaris*)	Worldwide	Primary amebic meningoencephalitis or granulomatous amebic encephalitis rarely involves the spine. May present with myelopathy commonly associated with brain lesions.	Solitary or multifocal, enhancing masslike lesions with peripheral edema, commonly associated with cerebritis.[57]

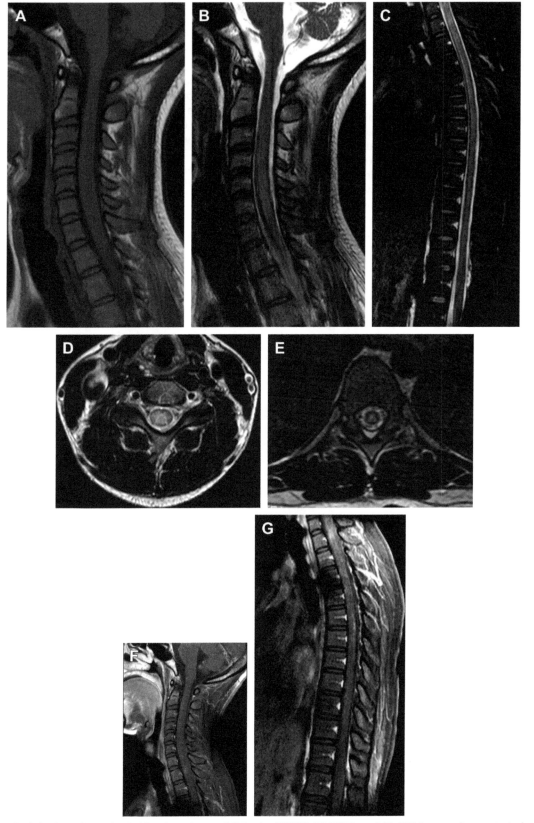

Fig. 13. Spinal cord Baggio-Yoshinari syndrome. (*A*) Sagittal T1WI, (*B*) T2WI, and (*C*) STIR images demonstrated a longitudinally extensive spinal cord lesion affecting almost the entire length. (*D, E*) Axial T2WI revealed predominant involvement of the gray matter, similar to spinal cord infarcts. (*F, G*) Sagittal fat-sat postcontrast T1WIs showed a subtle heterogeneous aspect to the spinal cord. There was also a mild leptomeningeal enhancement, characterized by a linear enhancement in the spinal cord surfaces.

enhancement on postcontrast T1WIs, especially in the facial nerve, may aid the diagnosis.[36–39]

Syphilis

Syphilis is a sexually transmissible disease caused by the spirochete *Treponema pallidum*. There has been a sharp increase in the number of cases of syphilis in the era of AIDS, with a corresponding increase in the incidence of neurologic disease.[8] The most common presentation of syphilis in the spine involves the presence of syphilitic gummas, which result from an intense leptomeningeal inflammatory reaction and may show the classic "candle guttering appearance" on contrast studies, as

well as the "flip-flop sign" characterized by low signal intensity on T2WIs and avid enhancement (Fig. 14). Another classic but currently rare presentation is *tabes dorsalis* (the tertiary form), which involves the posterior column of the spinal cord and can be demonstrated by nonspecific atrophy associated with hyperintensity on T2WIs.[8,40,41]

South American Blastomycosis (Paracoccidioidomycosis)

Overview

Paracoccidioidomycosis is a systemic disease caused by the dimorphic fungus *Paracoccidioides brasiliensis*. This disease predominates in South

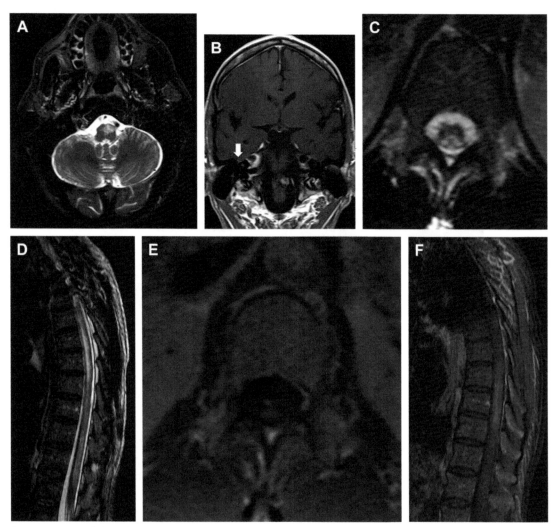

Fig. 14. Neurosyphilis. (*A*) Axial T2WI and (*B*) coronal postcontrast T1 images revealed a peripheral nodular lesion in the bulbo-medullary transition with an avid enhancement, consistent with a syphilitic gumma. Inner-ear structure enhancement was observed on the right side (*arrow*). (*C*) Axial T2WI and (*D*) sagittal STIR image demonstrated extensive perilesional vasogenic edema in the thoracic and lumbar spinal cord. (*E*) Axial and (*F*) sagittal fat-sat postcontrast T1WI showed an associated area of enhancement localized in the posterior aspect of the thoracic spinal cord, consistent with syphilitic myelitis.

America and therefore is also known as "South American blastomycosis."[42] It is the most important systemic profound mycosis in Latin America, especially in Brazil, where the prevalence in different regions has been reported to range from 5.6% to 17.5%. Rare cases have been reported in patients who have lived in or visited endemic areas.[8,42,43]

Pathophysiology
This disease occurs by inhalation of the fungus, with hematogenous or secondary lymphatic dissemination to the kidneys, spleen, adrenal glands, and bone, as well as CNS. This disease also has been recognized as an AIDS-related opportunistic infection in endemic areas.[5]

Diagnosis
Diagnostic confirmation is based on biopsy, usually outside the CNS. When paracoccidioidomycosis is suspected, a lung study, mainly using CT, is recommended for identifying the appropriate lesions for biopsy, particularly in the lung tissue.[8,42,43]

Imaging
CNS lesions may manifest as granulomas, meningitis, or as a mixed form. Localization in the spinal cord is considered rare, constituting only 0.6% of systemic infection cases and 4.0% when the CNS is involved.[42–44] CNS granulomas are lesions with an expanding aspect commonly associated with the involvement of other organs, most notably the lungs

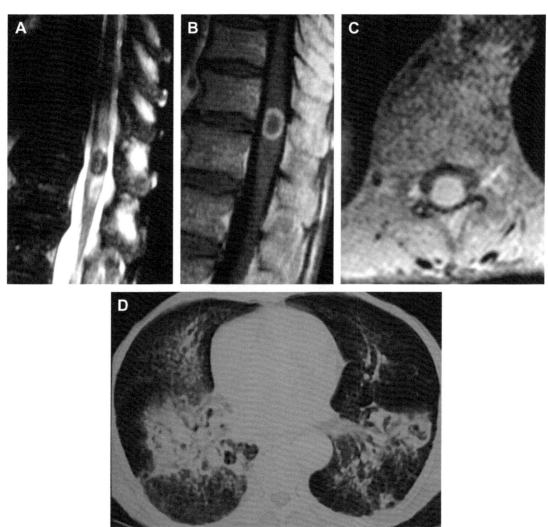

Fig. 15. Spinal cord paracoccidioidomycosis. The (A) sagittal STIR image, (B) postcontrast T1WI, and (C) axial fat-sat postcontrast T1WI demonstrated a focal nodular lesion in the medullary cone characterized by ring enhancement and T2 hypointensity with perilesional vasogenic edema. The imaging findings were not specific but suggested a granulomatous process. (D) A high-resolution lung CT scan revealed findings suggestive of paracoccidioidomycosis, including bilateral consolidations with associated multiple confluent nodules and interlobular septal thickening, more prominent in the central lung zone.

(Figs. 15 and 16).[42] These lesions also may be associated with diffuse leptomeningeal enhancement, characterizing the meningeal form.[45]

Human T-Lymphotropic Virus Type 1–Associated Myelopathy

Human T-lymphotropic virus type 1 (HTLV-1) infects 20 million individuals globally and is highly endemic in Japan and also prevalent in Melanesia, the Caribbean, and certain areas of Africa and Brazil.[46,47] This virus is transmitted through breast-feeding, blood transfusion, sexual intercourse, and intravenous drug use. Approximately 2% to 5% of patients will develop a progressive

myelopathy known as HTLV-1–associated myelopathy, which overlaps with tropical spastic paraparesis. These manifestations usually have a slow onset with chronic progression, and neurologic impairment develops within the first 2 years.[48] Punctate or confluent brain white matter lesions and spinal cord atrophy (74%) have been reported as MR findings of HTLV-1–associated myelopathy (Fig. 17).[47,49–51]

The progression of neurologic deficits can be accelerated (termed "acute HTLV-1–associated myelopathy") by a higher proviral load or previous blood transfusion, the involvement of extensive spinal cord lesions, which present as cord swelling, and vacuolation in the white matter.[47,48,52] These

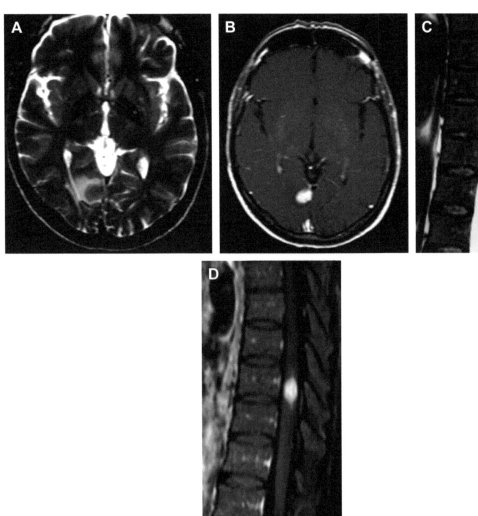

Fig. 16. Paracoccidioidomycosis. (A) Axial T2WI revealed a peripheral right occipital lobe hyperintense lesion. (B) The axial postcontrast T1WI showed nodular enhancement. The (C) sagittal STIR image and (D) sagittal fat-sat postcontrast T1WI demonstrated a similar lesion in the spinal cord associated with remarkable perilesional edema. (*Courtesy of* J.R. Ferraz, MD, Sao Jose do Rio Preto-SP, Brazil.)

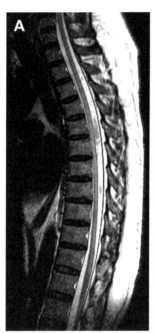
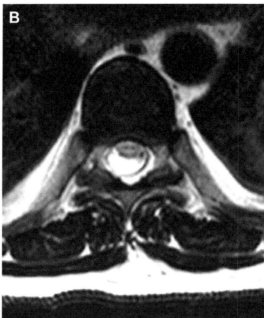

Fig. 17. HTLV-1–associated myelopathy (tropical spastic paraparesis). (*A*) Sagittal STIR image and (*B*) axial T2WI showed atrophy and an abnormal hyperintense signal affecting the entire spinal cord in a patient with HTLV-1–associated myelopathy. Note the incipient atrophy in the posterolateral areas of the spinal cord.

imaging findings resemble those described in neuromyelitis optica (NMO); moreover, some patients may present antibodies directed against the water channel aquaporin-4 antigen.[48] Nevertheless, acute HTLV-1–associated myelopathy and that associated with the NMO spectrum are distinct clinical entities; however, it is possible that HTLV-1 worsens the evolution and leads to a worse prognosis in patients with NMO.[46]

SUMMARY

As herein reported, radiologists play an important role in the early diagnosis and management of spinal parasitic diseases. MR imaging is very sensitive for characterizing the anatomic affected topography, providing accurate localization, characterizing the lesional pattern, delineating the associated changes, and monitoring the follow-up after therapy.

Thorough comprehension of the imaging features associated with the clinical features, epidemiology, laboratory results, and several imaging patterns of parasitic diseases allows the radiologist to narrow down the options for differential diagnosis and facilitate the timely implementation of appropriate therapies.

REFERENCES

1. DeSanto J, Ross JS. Spine infection/inflammation. Radiol Clin North Am 2011;49(1):105–27.

2. Abdel Razek AA, Watcharakorn A, Castillo M. Parasitic diseases of the central nervous system. Neuroimaging Clin N Am 2011;21(4):815–41, viii.

3. Quencer RM, Post MJ. Spinal cord lesions in patients with AIDS. Neuroimaging Clin N Am 1997;7(2):359–73.

4. Garcia HH, Gonzalez AE, Evans CA, et al, Cysticercosis Working Group in Peru. *Taenia solium* cysticercosis. Lancet 2003;362(9383):547–56.

5. do Amaral LL, Ferreira RM, da Rocha AJ, et al. Neurocysticercosis: evaluation with advanced magnetic resonance techniques and atypical forms. Top Magn Reson Imaging 2005;16(2):127–44.

6. Garcia HH, Del Brutto OH. *Taenia solium* cysticercosis. Infect Dis Clin North Am 2000;14(1):97–119, ix.

7. Del Brutto OH. Diagnostic criteria for neurocysticercosis, revisited. Pathog Glob Health 2012;106(5):299–304.

8. da Rocha AJ, Maia AC Jr, Ferreira NP, et al. Granulomatous diseases of the central nervous system. Top Magn Reson Imaging 2005;16(2):155–87.

9. Dumas JL, Visy JM, Belin C, et al. Parenchymal neurocysticercosis: follow-up and staging by MRI. Neuroradiology 1997;39(1):12–8.

10. Torabi AM, Quiceno M, Mendelsohn DB, et al. Multilevel intramedullary spinal neurocysticercosis with eosinophilic meningitis. Arch Neurol 2004;61(5):770–2.

11. Carod Artal FJ. Cerebral and spinal schistosomiasis. Curr Neurol Neurosci Rep 2012;12(6):666–74.

12. Ross AG, Bartley PB, Sleigh AC, et al. Schistosomiasis. N Engl J Med 2002;346(16):1212–20.

13. Jaureguiberry S, Paris L, Caumes E. Acute schistosomiasis, a diagnostic and therapeutic challenge. Clin Microbiol Infect 2010;16(3):225–31.

14. Ferrari TC, Moreira PR. Neuroschistosomiasis: clinical symptoms and pathogenesis. Lancet Neurol 2011;10(9):853–64.

15. Artal FJ, Mesquita HM, Gepp Rde A, et al. Neurological picture. Brain involvement in a Schistosoma mansoni myelopathy patient. J Neurol Neurosurg Psychiatry 2006;77(4):512.

16. Saleem S, Belal AI, El-Ghandour NM. Spinal cord schistosomiasis: MR imaging appearance with surgical and pathologic correlation. AJNR Am J Neuroradiol 2005;26(7):1646–54.

17. Sanelli PC, Lev MH, Gonzalez RG, et al. Unique linear and nodular MR enhancement pattern in schistosomiasis of the central nervous system: report of three patients. AJR Am J Roentgenol 2001;177(6):1471–4.

18. Ruberti RF, Saio M. Epidural Bilharzioma mansoni compressing the spinal cord: case report. East Afr Med J 1999;76(7):414–6.

19. Maia C Jr, Silva LR, Guimaraes MD, et al. Spinal cord compression secondary to epidural bilharzioma: case report. J Neuroimaging 2007;17(4):367–70.

20. Tuzun M, Hekimoglu B. Hydatid disease of the CNS: imaging features. AJR Am J Roentgenol 1998;171(6):1497–500.

21. Neumayr A, Tamarozzi F, Goblirsch S, et al. Spinal cystic echinococcosis–a systematic analysis and review of the literature: part 1. Epidemiology and anatomy. PLoS Negl Trop Dis 2013;7(9):e2450.

22. Czermak BV, Unsinn KM, Gotwald T, et al. Echinococcus granulosus revisited: radiologic patterns seen in pediatric and adult patients. AJR Am J Roentgenol 2001;177(5):1051–6.

23. Polat P, Kantarci M, Alper F, et al. Hydatid disease from head to toe. Radiographics 2003;23(2):475–94 [quiz: 536–7].

24. Jongwutiwes U, Yanagida T, Ito A, et al. Isolated intradural-extramedullary spinal cysticercosis: a case report. J Travel Med 2011;18(4):284–7.

25. Montoya JG, Liesenfeld O. Toxoplasmosis. Lancet 2004;363(9425):1965–76.

26. Mohle L, Parlog A, Pahnke J, et al. Spinal cord pathology in chronic experimental Toxoplasma gondii infection. Eur J Microbiol Immunol (Bp) 2014;4(1):65–75.

27. Maciel E, Siqueira I, Queiroz AC, et al. Toxoplasma gondii myelitis in a patient with adult T-cell leukemia-lymphoma. Arq Neuropsiquiatr 2000;58(4):1107–9.

28. Rodgers J. Trypanosomiasis and the brain. Parasitology 2010;137(14):1995–2006.

29. Jackson Y, Chappuis F. Chagas disease in Switzerland: history and challenges. Euro Surveill 2011;16(37) [pii:19963].

30. Lury KM, Castillo M. Chagas' disease involving the brain and spinal cord: MRI findings. AJR Am J Roentgenol 2005;185(2):550–2.

31. Finsterer J, Auer H. Parasitoses of the human central nervous system. J Helminthol 2013;87(3):257–70.

32. Juncos RA, Abdala J. Chagasic myelitis. Rev Fac Cienc Med Cordoba 1960;18:123–7 [in Spanish].

33. Steere AC. Lyme disease. N Engl J Med 2001;345(2):115–25.

34. Yoshinari NH, Mantovani E, Bonoldi VL, et al. Brazilian lyme-like disease or Baggio-Yoshinari syndrome: exotic and emerging Brazilian tick-borne zoonosis. Rev Assoc Med Bras 2010;56(3):363–9 [in Portuguese].

35. Shinjo SK, Gauditano G, Marchiori PE, et al. Manifestação neurologica na Sindrome de Baggio-Yoshinari. Rev Bras Reumatol 2009;49:492–505.

36. Vanzieleghem B, Lemmerling M, Carton D, et al. Lyme disease in a child presenting with bilateral facial nerve palsy: MRI findings and review of the literature. Neuroradiology 1998;40(11):739–42.

37. Hattingen E, Weidauer S, Kieslich M, et al. MR imaging in neuroborreliosis of the cervical spinal cord. Eur Radiol 2004;14(11):2072–5.

38. Fernandez RE, Rothberg M, Ferencz G, et al. Lyme disease of the CNS: MR imaging findings in 14 cases. AJNR Am J Neuroradiol 1990;11(3):479–81.

39. Rocha AJ, Littig IA, Nunes RH, et al. Central nervous system infectious diseases mimicking multiple sclerosis: recognizing distinguishable features using MRI. Arq Neuropsiquiatr 2013;71(9B):738–46.

40. He D, Jiang B. Syphilitic myelitis: magnetic resonance imaging features. Neurol India 2014;62(1):89–91.

41. Tashiro K, Moriwaka F, Sudo K, et al. Syphilitic myelitis with its magnetic resonance imaging (MRI) verification and successful treatment. Jpn J Psychiatry Neurol 1987;41(2):269–71.

42. de Almeida SM. Central nervous system paracoccidioidomycosis: an overview. Braz J Infect Dis 2005;9(2):126–33.

43. Colli BO, Assirati Junior JA, Machado HR, et al. Intramedullary spinal cord paracoccidioidomycosis. Report of two cases. Arq Neuropsiquiatr 1996;54(3):466–73.

44. de Moura LP, Raffin CN, del Negro GM, et al. Paracoccidioidomycosis evidencing spinal cord involvement treated with success by fluconazole. Arq Neuropsiquiatr 1994;52(1):82–6 [in Portuguese].

45. Lorenzoni PJ, Chang MR, Paniago AM, et al. Paracoccidioidomycosis meningitis: case report. Arq Neuropsiquiatr 2002;60(4):1015–8 [in Portuguese].

46. von Glehn FC, Casseb J, Brandao CO, et al. Distinguishing characteristics between transverse myelitis associated with neuromyelitis optica and HTIV-1-associated myelopathy. Latin American Multiple Sclerosis Journal 2013;2(1):24–9.

47. Shakudo M, Inoue Y, Tsutada T. HTLV-I-associated myelopathy: acute progression and atypical MR findings. AJNR Am J Neuroradiol 1999;20(8): 1417–21.

48. Delgado SR, Sheremata WA, Brown AD, et al. Human T-lymphotropic virus type I or II (HTLV-I/II) associated with recurrent longitudinally extensive transverse myelitis (LETM): two case reports. J Neurovirol 2010;16(3):249–53.

49. Alcindor F, Valderrama R, Canavaggio M, et al. Imaging of human T-lymphotropic virus type I-associated chronic progressive myeloneuropathies. Neuroradiology 1992;35(1):69–74.

50. Godoy AJ, Kira J, Hasuo K, et al. Characterization of cerebral white matter lesions of HTLV-I-associated myelopathy/tropical spastic paraparesis in comparison with multiple sclerosis and collagen-vasculitis: a semiquantitative MRI study. J Neurol Sci 1995; 133(1–2):102–11.

51. Melo A, Moura L, Rios S, et al. Magnetic resonance imaging in HTLV-I associated myelopathy. Arq Neuropsiquiatr 1993;51(3):329–32.

52. Araujo AQ, Silva MT. The HTLV-1 neurological complex. Lancet Neurol 2006;5(12):1068–76.

53. Mani S, Mondal SS, Guha G, et al. Acute disseminated encephalomyelitis after mixed malaria infection (Plasmodium falciparum and Plasmodium vivax) with MRI closely simulating multiple sclerosis. Neurologist 2011;17(5):276–8.

54. Kibiki GS, Murphy DK. Transverse myelitis due to trypanosomiasis in a middle aged Tanzanian man. J Neurol Neurosurg Psychiatry 2006;77(5):684–5.

55. Lee IH, Kim ST, Oh DK, et al. MRI findings of spinal visceral larva migrans of Toxocara canis. Eur J Radiol 2010;75(2):236–40.

56. Lin J, Arita JH, da Rocha AJ, et al. Enlarging the spectrum of inflammatory/post-infectious acute disseminated encephalomyelitis: a further case associated with neurotoxocariasis. J Neuroparasitology 2010;1:1–3.

57. Viriyavejakul P, Rochanawutanon M, Sirinavin S. Naegleria meningomyeloencephalitis. Southeast Asian J Trop Med Public Health 1997;28(1):237–40.

Image Guided Interventions in Spinal Infections

Prof Massimo Gallucci, MD[a],*, Federico D'Orazio, MD[b]

KEYWORDS

- Spinal infections • Image guided interventions • Computed tomography-guided biopsies
- Percutaneous drainage of the spine

KEY POINTS

- The diagnosis of spinal infection is still today a challenging exercise; it can need one or more spine biopsies before the causative agent is isolated from specimens.
- To perform spine biopsies, there are several image-guidance available technologies, such as fluoroscopy, computed tomography, and MR imaging.
- Depending on the level of spine which is involved, a different approach and positioning of the patient should be used by the interventional radiologist.
- Antibiotic therapies eventually administered before the biopsy is performed can represent a main confounding factor; in those cases the sensitivity of the biopsy itself is further decreased.
- Percutaneous drainage of inflammatory collections eventually associated with spinal infections represents a safe and minimally invasive method to rapidly treat complications of spinal infections and can also be used to administer locally antibiotics.

INTRODUCTION

The diagnosis of spinal infections is still today a challenging exercise, and it can need one or more spine biopsies before the causative agent can be isolated from specimens. Imaging findings are rather characteristic, if compared to those associated with malignancy of the spine, but when facing cases with advanced pathology, it can be more difficult to assess the true nature of a process that can produce extensive disruption of spine components and their surrounding tissues.

Diagnosis can be difficult and is often delayed because of the nonspecific accompanying symptoms.

The role of interventional neuroradiology in spinal infection is double: diagnostic and therapeutic, consisting substantially of 2 main procedures, represented by spine biopsies and positioning of percutaneous drainage, which represent a minimally invasive, faster and more cost-effective alternative to open surgery procedures proposed for the same purposes.

This article will focus on the available techniques to perform discovertebral image-guided biopsies in case of suspected infections and on image-guided placement of percutaneous drainage to treat infectious collections of the spine and paravertebral structures.

Disclosures: The Authors declare they have nothing to disclose.
[a] Neuroradiology Unit, S. Salvatore Hospital, University of L'Aquila, Via L. Natali, L'Aquila 67100, Italy;
[b] Neuroradiology Unit, S. Salvatore Hospital, Via L. Natali, L'Aquila 67100, Italy
* Corresponding author.
E-mail address: massimo.gallucci@cc.univaq.it

Clinical cases from the personal experience will be reported, analyzing the imaging characteristics that lead one to formulate suspicion of spinal infection, with the interventional treatment adopted and follow-up evaluation.

A major focus will be applied on computed tomography (CT)-guided discovertebral biopsies, which represent a more diffuse way to perform safely and quickly spine biopsies in several pathologies of this anatomic district.

SPINE BIOPSIES

Before proceeding with a biopsy of the spine, it is necessary to perform or review the radiological examinations that have raised its demand; these can be plain film radiographs, CT or MR imaging studies. The latter are usually preferred because of their higher sensitivity and specificity in detecting lesions of the spine and are often necessary to assess potentially associated spinal cord lesions of the involved spine tract.

The biopsy itself can be performed under several imaging guidances, such as fluoroscopy, CT and MR imaging; MR imaging-guided procedures are not yet widespread because of the costs and time spent to perform interventional procedures that, with the present technology, can be made more quickly and with superimposable safety under CT guidance, limiting significantly the radiation dose to which both patient and operator are exposed.

Fluoroscopy can represent an easy guidance method, but cannot show all the anatomic structures to be preserved during the procedure (ie, mainly nerve roots and vessels).

In case of multiple spine lesions, it is advisable to proceed to biopsy the level with fewer potential complications and with greater chances of easy and less traumatic percutaneous access.

Preparation

The patient must not drink or eat for a minimum of 8 hours prior to the procedure; it is necessary to acquire some important laboratory parameters to asses coagulation profile (prothrombin time [PT], partial thromboplastin time [PTT], international normalized ratio [INR]) and eventual allergies to drugs, especially local anesthetics and contrast media.

The procedure is often performed with a combination of local anesthetic (usually bupivacaine 1%) and intravenous conscious sedation using benzodiazepine. If a vertebral body has to be entered, the administration of local anesthetics around the periosteum is helpful to minimize the discomfort associated with the procedure.

Patient Positioning

Patient positioning depends on the level where the spinal biopsy is proposed; a prone position is often preferable for thoracic and lumbar lesions. In the case of a cervical lesion, a supine position is requested to gain anterolateral access to the cervical spinal tract; prone positioning should be considered safe to perform biopsy of the posterior cervical arches.

Depending on the patient clinical conditions, sometimes it is necessary to proceed to biopsy with an oblique prone or lateral decubitus.

Technique of Specimen Acquisition

There are 2 main possibilities that are almost always used together when performing a spine biopsy: aspiration biopsy and core biopsy.

Aspiration biopsy requires smaller caliber needles (18–22 G), while to perform core biopsy, greater cutting needles or bone biopsy needles are requested (10–14G); in the latter case, a small sample of tissue can be sent to pathologic examination, while the first method is more often preferred to produce specimens for microbiological analysis; actually, nothing prevents one from proceeding with aspiration through the same core biopsy needle used before.

These needles can be used with a tandem or coaxial technique.

Once the specimens have been acquired, to perform microbiological analysis, they must be placed in sterile containers and immediately sent to the laboratory; in case of aspiration biopsies it is of frequent observation the presence of blood, especially when the aspiration is performed after a core biopsy. It is important to consider that not only the frustules coming from the biopsy core site can be useful for microbiological or cytologic analysis, but also blood can be used for diagnostic purposes; thus it should not be considered as a waste and useless material. When multiple biopsy passes are performed and, if it is needed to rule out in differential diagnosis malignancy, part of

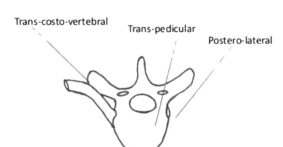

Fig. 1. Percutaneous ways of access to vertebrae.

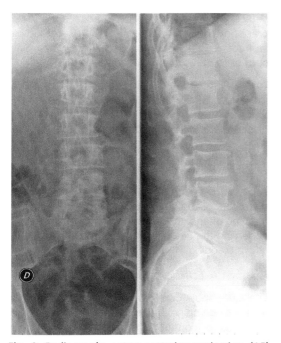

Fig. 2. Radiograph; anteroposterior projection (AP) and laterolateral projection (LL) view. Degenerative changes in the presacral space, with slight thickening of the limiting somatic of L4 and L5 vertebral body.

the specimens can be put in containers with formalin 10% and sent to the pathology laboratory.

Tandem technique

This technique involves the use of 2 distinct needles; the first and smaller needle is used to administer local anesthetics alongside the trajectory planned for biopsy; once used, it is left in place to serve as a visual guide.

Coaxial technique

The localizing cannula is used to administrate local anesthetics and as a mechanical guide for the biopsy needle, which is coaxial to the cannula; using this technique, several passes with the biopsy needle are possible through the cannula, with major possibilities of diagnostic results and minor complication rates.

Percutaneous Approach to the Spine

The main determining factors to choose the way of percutaneous approach to the spine are represented by the lesion level and its dimensions.

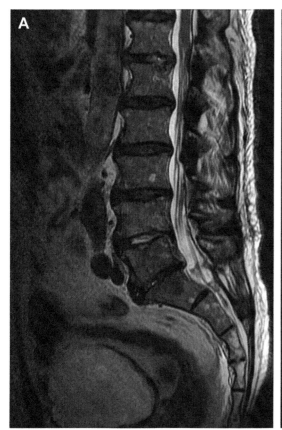
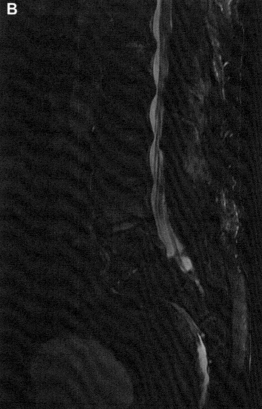

Fig. 3. (A) MR imaging sagittal plane, T2 weighted image. Bright signal of the intervertebral disc L4–L5. (B) MR imaging sagittal plane, T2 weighted image with fat suppression. Bone marrow edema in L4–L5.

The anterolateral approach is preferable only in the case of anterior cervical lesions; it requires great skills and experience as well as manual displacement of the neurovascular bundle of the neck. Otherwise, posterior access is safer in case of posterior cervical, thoracic, and lumbosacral lesions.

For thoracic biopsies, it is good practice to perform biopsies using a right lateral access, to avoid accidental injury to the aorta.

Posterior approach

Three ways of posterior approach can be distinguished (**Fig. 1**).

Posterolateral This approach is useful for lesions located within the vertebral body, intervertebral disc, or paraspinal tissues; it is clearly the most often used for biopsies in suspected spinal infections.

Transpedicular This approach is used to access inside thoracic and lumbar vertebral bodies. The pedicle provides a safe way to access the vertebral body, but great care must be used to avoid its fracture, which can cause injury to the spinal cord or to the exiting spinal nerve root.

Trans-costo-vertebral This approach is used only for lesions of the thoracic tract; it allows to one to reach the vertebral body, the intervertebral disc, and the paraspinal thoracic structures.

Postoperative Care

Immediately after the procedure, a sterile dressing is placed over the entry site(s). Patients must be observed for the next 2 to 4 hours, depending on the type of anesthesia used during the procedure, observing the site of access for eventual signs of active bleeding.

Diagnostic Efficacy

Literature show conflicting data about diagnostic reliability of spine biopsies in spinal infections, but it is a common consideration that spine

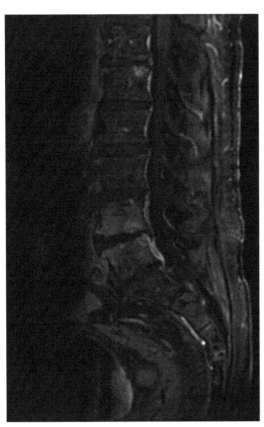

Fig. 4. MR imaging sagittal plane, T1 weighted image with fat suppression + Gd. After gadolinium administration inhomogeneous bone marrow enhancement is seen.

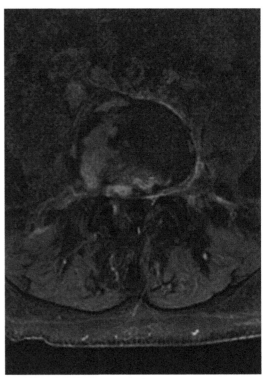

Fig. 5. MR imaging axial plane, T1 weighted images with fat suppression + Gd. After gadolinium administration, bone marrow enhancement is seen together with some slight enhancement of the paravertebral structures and initial epidural collection posterior to L5 vertebral body.

biopsies, when made to diagnose spinal infections, have lesser diagnostic power than those performed in case of either primitive and secondary malignancy, and they are commonly reported to have positive results in a percentage varying between 15% to 70% of cases, depending also on the caliber of the needles used to perform such procedures.[1–5] Actually, the most important factor influencing this result is surely represented by the fact that often patients with suspected spinal infections have already been under antibiotic therapy for several days.[6–8] In such cases, it is possible to repeat the biopsy after at least 1 week without antibiotic therapy, and in those cases, literature data homogeneously show higher diagnostic power of the biopsies repeated after this measure.[9–12]

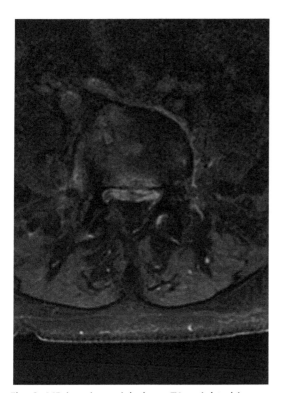

Fig. 6. MR imaging axial plane, T1 weighted images with fat suppression + Gd. After gadolinium administration, bone marrow enhancement is seen together with some slight enhancement of the paravertebral structures and initial epidural collection posterior to L5 vertebral body.

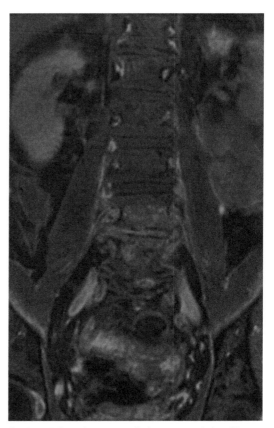

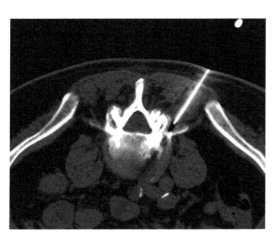

Fig. 7. CT scan. Spine biopsy of the L5 vertebral body is performed with posterior transpedicular approach.

Fig. 8. MR imaging coronal plane, T1 weighted image with fat suppression + Gd. At the 3 weeks later control MR imaging, after gadolinium administration an extended granulation tissue at the L4–L5 tract is seen, with reduction of the inflammatory collection previously observed.

PERCUTANEOUS DRAINAGE
When It Is Necessary?

Placement of a percutaneous drainage is requested to rapidly remove large fluid inflammatory collections that can be associated with advanced phases of spinal infections, to reduce local inflammation, and accelerate healing of the infection itself; they can be used also to introduce directly in situ antibiotics and produce materials for microbiological testing.

Technique

Once the level of the collection and its anatomic relationships with the nearest structures to be preserved have been identified, the drainage is placed using the same tricks and techniques used for

biopsy and exposed earlier; it is almost always used a posterolateral approach to reach the collection, which can affect the psoas muscles and/or other minor paravertebral muscles.

The same precautions taken for the execution of spine biopsies must be taken in account for placement of a drainage (ie, evaluation of coagulation parameters and allergies).

6–8 F drainage catheters can be used, and they are more safely placed using CT guidance. Great care has to be used to avoid the nearest structures that could be damaged while inserting the drainage catheter. Once positioned, the catheter can be connected to an airtight bag or a container with internal negative pressure so as to ensure continuous aspiration.

Once the collection is resolved and the antibiotics have been injected locally, the drainage can be safely removed.

CLINICAL CASES
Case Number 1

A 74-year-old man presented with low back pain for 3 weeks without history of previous trauma.

First radiograph examination (**Fig. 2**) showed mild degenerative phenomena on L4-L5 and L5-S1 spaces; 3 weeks later, because of worsening symptoms with same location and fever (39°C) an MR imaging of lumbosacral tract was performed, showing (**Fig. 3**) bone marrow edema

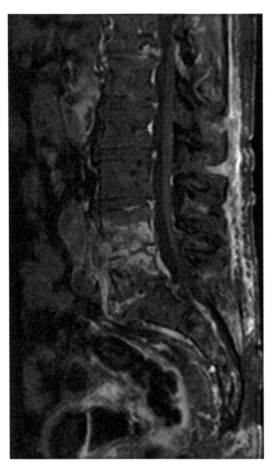

Fig. 9. MR imaging sagittal plane, T1 weighted image with fat suppression + Gd. At the 3 weeks later control MR imaging, after gadolinium administration an extended granulation tissue at the L4–L5 tract is seen, with reduction of the inflammatory collection previously observed.

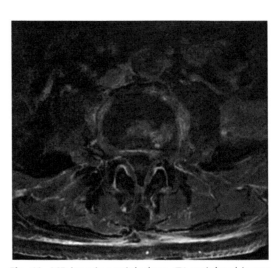

Fig. 10. MR imaging axial plane, T1 weighted image with fat suppression + Gd. At the 3 weeks later control MR imaging, after gadolinium administration an extended granulation tissue at the L4–L5 tract is seen, with reduction of the inflammatory collection previously observed.

of L4 and L5 vertebral bodies and bright signal of the intervertebral disc. After administration of gadolinium (**Figs. 4** and **5**), inhomogeneous contrast enhancement is seen, with appearance of small amount of epidural abscess behind L5 (**Fig. 6**). Immediately after, a CT-guided spine biopsy was performed at L5, with a transpedicular approach (**Fig. 7**). Spondylodiscitis sustained by *Staphylococcus aureus* was demonstrated after microbiological examination of the specimens.

Three weeks later, with slight improvement of symptoms, a control MR imaging (**Figs. 8–10**) showed extended granulation tissue at the L4–L5 tract, with reduction of the inflammatory collection previously seen. Ten months later, new a control MR imaging showed normalization of findings (**Figs. 11–14**).

Case Number 2

A 70-year-old presented with colon cancer and rapidly worsening dorsal pain but no history of previous trauma. The patient had acute weakness of lower limbs and a history of pulmonary tuberculosis in youth.

First MR imaging examination was performed for suspect pathologic dorsal fracture (ie, bony metastasis from colon cancer) and showed extensive deformity of the dorsal tract T6–T8 determining displacement of the spinal cord associated to bone marrow edema with paravertebral fluid collections (**Figs. 15–19**); after gadolinium intravenous injection extensive and intense enhancement of both vertebrae, discs, and fluid collections walls was seen, with signs of local meningeal reaction. The same day, a CT-guided

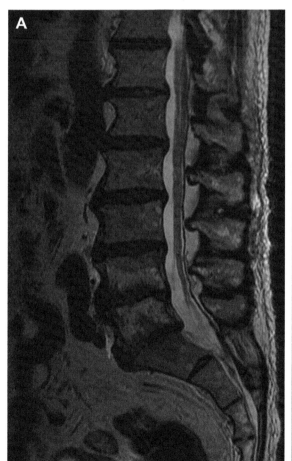
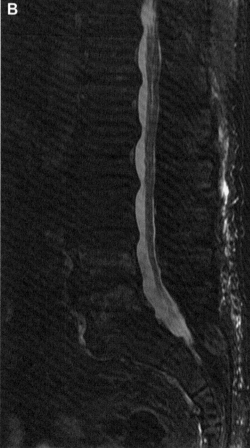

Fig. 11. (*A*) MR imaging sagittal plane, T2 weighted image. (*B*) MR imaging sagittal plane, T2 weighted image with fat suppression. At the 10-month MR imaging follow-up, a normalization of the findings was shown, with almost complete disappearance of the bone marrow enhancement, and complete resolution of the fluid collections.

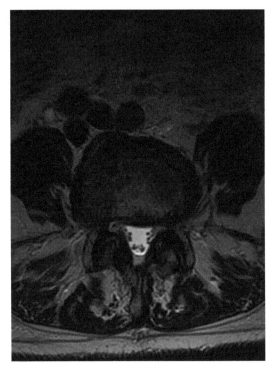

Fig. 12. MR imaging axial plane, T2 weighted image. At the 10 month MR imaging follow-up, a normalization of the findings was shown, with almost complete disappearance of the bone marrow enhancement, and complete resolution of the fluid collections.

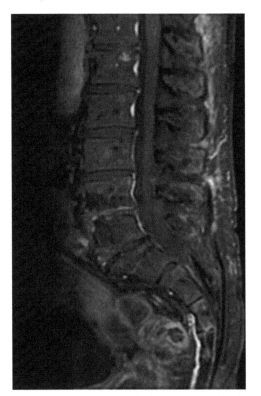

Fig. 13. MR imaging sagittal plane, T1 weighted image with fat suppression + Gd. At the 10-month MR imaging follow-up, a normalization of the findings was shown, with almost complete disappearance of the bone marrow enhancement, and complete resolution of the fluid collections.

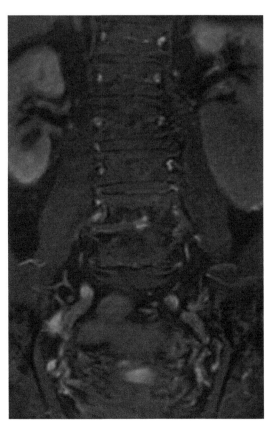

Fig. 14. Coronal plane, T1 weighted image with fat suppression + Gd. At the 10-month MR imaging follow-up, a normalization of the findings was shown, with almost complete disappearance of the bone marrow enhancement, and complete resolution of the fluid collections.

biopsy and aspiration of the collections were scheduled. The preliminary CT scan (**Figs. 20**) showed wide lytic bone phenomena. The biopsy was performed with a trans-costo-vertebral approach (**Fig. 21**), and aspiration of the fluid paravertebral collections was performed with a posterolateral approach (**Fig. 22**). Spondylodiscitis sustained by *Mycobacterium tuberculosis* will be found on examination of the fluid collection.

Three weeks later, control MR imaging showed slight reduction of bone marrow edema (**Fig. 23**), disappearance of the collections, and spinal cord displacement, with persistent intense enhancement of the bony structures (**Figs. 24** and **25**).

Case Number 3

An 80-year-old man Presented with lung cancer and recurrence of pulmonary tuberculosis, Fever and intense low back pain, and paraplegia. MR

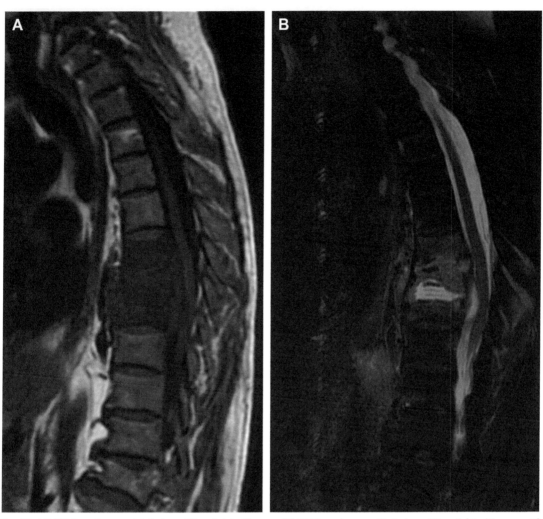

Fig. 15. (*A*) MR imaging, sagittal plane, T1 weighted image. (*B*) MR imaging, sagittal plane, T2 weighted image with fat suppression. Large involvement of the T6–T8 thoracic tract of the spine, with involvement of the intervertebral discs, fluid collections in the paravertebral tissues, and displacement of the spinal cord by mean of an epidural abscess.

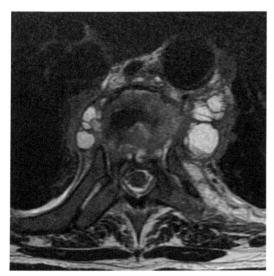

Fig. 16. MR imaging, axial plane, T2 weighted image. Large involvement of the T6–T8 thoracic tract of the spine, with involvement of the intervertebral discs, fluid collections in the paravertebral tissues, and displacement of the spinal cord by mean of an epidural abscess.

imaging examinations showed an important deformity of the L2–L4 tract of spine (**Fig. 26**). Preliminary CT scan showed wide lytic phenomena involving the vertebral bodies (**Fig. 27**) with some fluid collections. A biopsy was performed subsequently with a posterolateral approach (**Fig. 28**); using the same approach, a drainage was placed (**Figs. 29** and **30**).

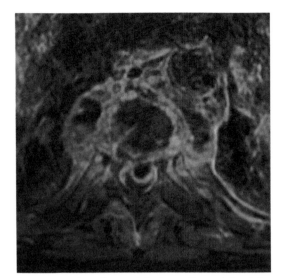

Fig. 17. MR imaging, axial plane, T1 weighted image + Gd. Large involvement of the T6–T8 thoracic tract of the spine, with involvement of the intervertebral discs, fluid collections in the paravertebral tissues and displacement of the spinal cord by mean of an epidural abscess.

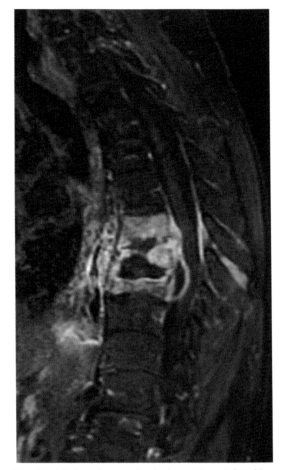

Fig. 19. MR imaging, sagittal plane, T1 weighted image + Gd. Large involvement of the T6–T8 thoracic tract of the spine, with involvement of the intervertebral discs, fluid collections in the paravertebral tissues, and displacement of the spinal cord by mean of an epidural abscess.

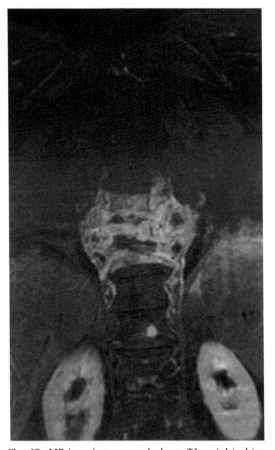

Fig. 18. MR imaging, coronal plane, T1 weighted image + Gd. Large involvement of the T6–T8 thoracic tract of the spine, with involvement of the intervertebral discs, fluid collections in the paravertebral tissues, and displacement of the spinal cord by mean of an epidural abscess.

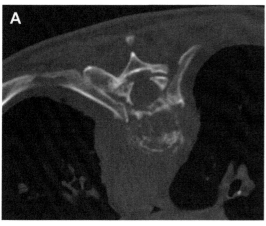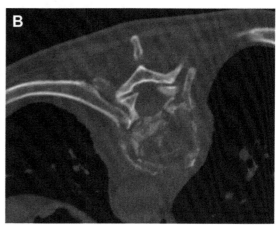

Fig. 20. (*A*, *B*) CT scan. Lytic changes of the vertebral bodies with paravertebral fluid mass around thoracic aorta.

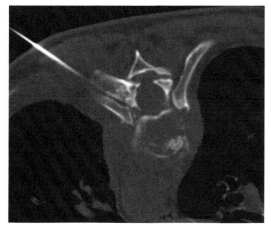

Fig. 21. CT scan. CT-guided biopsy is performed with posterior trans-costo-vertebral approach.

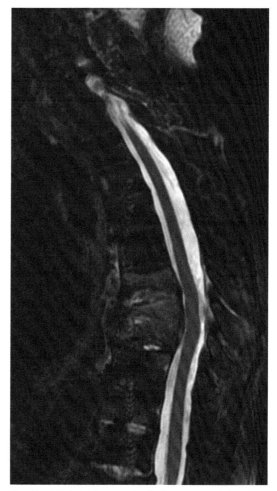

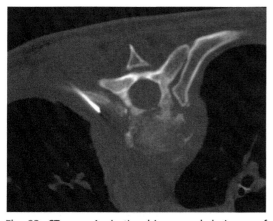

Fig. 22. CT scan. Aspiration biopsy and drainage of the fluid paravertebral collections is made under CT guidance, with posterolateral approach.

Fig. 23. MR imaging, sagittal plane, T2 weighted image with fat suppression. At the 3 week control MR imaging follow-up, disappearance of the fluid paravertebral and epidural collection was seen, with persistent intense enhancement of the vertebral bodies on paravertebral tissues.

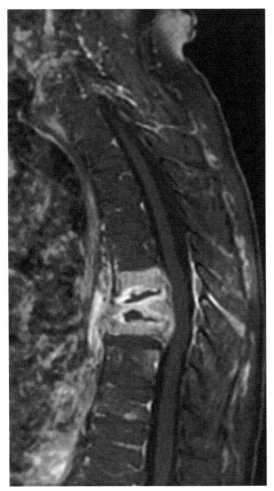

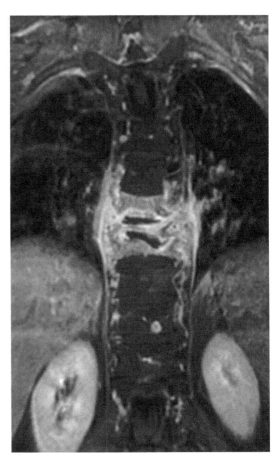

Fig. 24. MR imaging, sagittal plane, T1 weighted image with fat suppression + Gd. At the 3-weeks control MR imaging, disappearance of the fluid paravertebral and epidural collection was seen, with persistent intense enhancement of the vertebral bodies on paravertebral tissues.

Fig. 25. MR imaging, coronal plane, T1 weighted image with fat suppression + Gd. At the 3-week control MR imaging follow-up, disappearance of the fluid paravertebral and epidural collection was seen, with persistent intense enhancement of the vertebral bodies on paravertebral tissues.

SUMMARY

Spine biopsies can be performed using several imaging methods (fluoroscopy, MR imaging, or CT), but with the current technologies, CT-guided spine biopsies are the gold standard for the diagnosis of spondilodiskitis and other forms of spinal/paraspinal infectious diseases. They allow diagnosis and first-line treatment of some associated conditions, such as epidural or paravertebral abscesses drainage, which can be helpful to increase overall survival of this potentially life-threatening medical condition.

Previous antibiotic therapy administration has been recognized as a major cause for negative results of microbiological examination of the specimens obtained; when this happens, it is advisable to repeat biopsy some days after suspension of the antibiotic therapy.

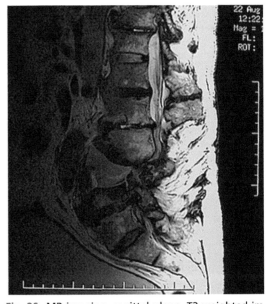

Fig. 26. MR imaging, sagittal plane, T2 weighted image. Extensive deformity of the L2–L4 tract of the lumbar spine with involvement of the intervertebral discs, which appear extensively damaged.

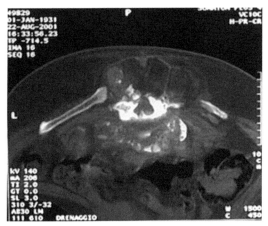

Fig. 27. CT scan. Extensive lytic lesions of the vertebral body with some fluid collections in the prevertebral space.

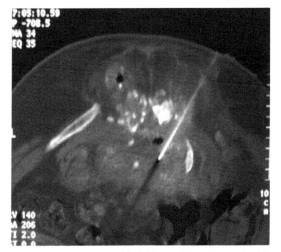

Fig. 28. CT scan. CT-guided biopsy is performed with posterolateral approach.

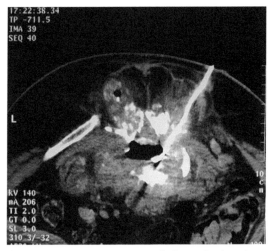

Fig. 29. CT scan. Percutaneous drainage is placed under CT guidance immediately after spine biopsy, with same posterolateral approach.

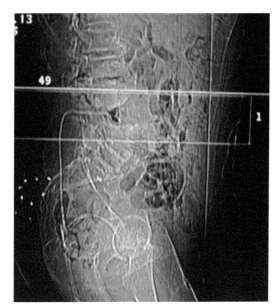

Fig. 30. CT scanogram, LL view. A drainage was placed and connected to a sac.

Observing simple good practice rules, CT-guided biopsy can be considered a safe, minimally invasive, and effective method to diagnose spine infections.

REFERENCES

1. Sehn JK, Gilula LA. Percutaneous needle biopsy in diagnosis and identification of causative organisms in cases of suspected vertebral osteomyelitis. Eur J Radiol 2012;81:940–6.
2. Tehranzadeh J, Tao C, Browning CA. Percutaneous needle biopsy of the spine. Acta Radiol 2007;48:860–8.
3. Chew FS, Kline MJ. Diagnostic yield of CT-guided percutaneous aspiration procedures in suspected spontaneous infectious diskitis. Radiology 2001;218:211–4.
4. Nourbakhsh A, Grady JJ, Garges KJ. Percutaneous spine biopsy: a meta-analysis. J Bone Joint Surg Am 2008;90:1722–5.
5. Phadke DM, Lucas DR, Madan S. Fine-needle aspiration biopsy of vertebral and intervertebral disc lesions: specimen adequacy, diagnostic utility, and pitfalls. Arch Pathol Lab Med 2001;125:1463–8.
6. Michel SC, Pfirrmann CW, Boos N, et al. CT-guided core biopsy of subchondral bone and intervertebral space in suspected Spondylodiscitis. AJR Am J Roentgenol 2006;186:977–80.
7. Rankine JJ, Barron DA, Robinson P, et al. Therapeutic impact of percutaneous spinal biopsy in spinal infection. Postgrad Med J 2004;80:607–9.

8. Wirtz DC, Genius I, Wildberger JE, et al. Diagnostic and therapeutic management of lumbar and thoracic spondylodiscitis—an evaluation of 59 cases. Arch Orthop Trauma Surg 2000;120:245–51.

9. Hau MA, Kim JI, Kattapuram S, et al. Accuracy of CT-guided biopsies in 359 patients with musculoskeletal lesions. Skeletal Radiol 2002;31:349–53.

10. De Lucas EM, Mandly AG, Gutierrez A, et al. CT-guided fine-needle aspiration in vertebral osteomyelitis: true usefulness of a common practice. Clin Rheumatol 2009;28:315–20.

11. Enoch DA, Cargill JS, Laing R, et al. Value of CT-guided biopsy in the diagnosis of septic discitis. J Clin Pathol 2008;61:750–3.

12. Yang SC, Chen WJ, Chen HS, et al. Extended indications of percutaneous endoscopic lavage and drainage for the treatment of lumbar infectious spondylitis. Eur Spine J 2014;23:846–53.

Neurosurgical Approaches to Spinal Infections

Derya Burcu Hazer, MD[a], Selim Ayhan, MD[b],
Selcuk Palaoglu, MD, PhD[c],*

KEYWORDS

• Spine • Infection • Surgery • Postoperative infection • Instability • Decompression • Deformity

KEY POINTS

• Spinal infections may be life threatening.
• Surgery is indicated in inadequate biopsies, conservative treatment failure, neurologic deterioration, spinal instability and deformity.
• In abrupt neurologic deterioration, emergency surgery must be performed.
• Choice of the operative procedure depends on the causative agent, site of the lesion, neurologic status, and bone destruction.

INTRODUCTION

Spinal infections are rare pathologies that compromise 2% to 4% of all bone infections.[1,2] These infections often jeopardize both the integrity of the spinal column and its neural contents, creating a consumptive process that may be life threatening. Therefore, in recent years more attention has been paid to spinal infections with the availability of increased diagnostic accuracy. Yet, even with improved diagnostic tools and procedures, delays in diagnosis remains an important issue.[3] Spinal infections can be categorized according to the different entities, such as contagious agent, anatomic localization, and onset of disease. There is usually also a predisposing factor that compromises the immune system and affects the spread as well as the severity of disease. Postoperative spinal infections are an important topic. Management of spinal infections requires a multidisciplinary approach involving spinal surgeons, infectious disease specialists, radiologists, rehabilitation personnel, psychologists, and social services. We emphasize neurosurgical approaches to spinal infections, focusing on anatomic location and causative agent.

NORMAL ANATOMY

Spinal infections are located mainly in the epidural space, body of the vertebra, intervertebral disc, perivertebral area, and intradural space. Infection may be localized in one of these compartments. Erosion of vertebral endplates causes deformation of the cortical lining and spreads to disc space (spondylodiscitis), subligamentous paravertebral space (paravertebral and psoas abscesses), and/or epidural–intradural space (epidural abscesses, intradural abscesses, and meningitis), consecutively.

The authors certify that there is no conflict of interest with any financial organization regarding the material discussed in the article.
[a] Department of Neurosurgery, Mugla Sitki Kocman University School of Medicine, Orhaniye Mahallesi, Haluk Ozsoy Caddesi, Mugla 48000, Turkey; [b] Malatya State Hospital, Department of Neurosurgery, Firat Mahallesi, Hastane Caddesi, Malatya 44330, Turkey; [c] Department of Neurosurgery, Hacettepe University School of Medicine, Sihhiye, Altindag, Ankara 06100, Turkey
* Corresponding author.
E-mail address: palaoglu@gmail.com

Neuroimag Clin N Am 25 (2015) 295–308
http://dx.doi.org/10.1016/j.nic.2015.01.008
1052-5149/15/$ – see front matter © 2015 Elsevier Inc. All rights reserved.

PATHOLOGY

The spine is known to be susceptible to infections with the incidence varies between 1:100,000 and 1:250,000 in developed countries. According to the literature, mortality rate ranges between 2% and 17%.[4,5] There is a superiority in males and age distribution has 2 peaks: under age 20 and between age 50 and 70.[4,6]

The major causative agents of spine infections are bacteria, which cause pyogenic infections; tuberculosis (TB) or fungi, which are responsible for granulomatous infections; and parasites, which are the least common etiology. Among them, the majority are bacterial pyogenic infections owing to *Staphylococcus aureus*.[7] Of note, in one-third of all cases of spinal infections, the infectious agent could not be identified.[8]

Pathogen spread occurs via 3 routes: hematogenous, direct external inoculation (iatrogenic), and spread from contiguous tissues. Risk factors for spinal infections include previous spine surgery, distant infectious foci, diabetes mellitus, malnutrition, advanced age, intravenous drug abuse, human immunodeficiency virus infection, a history of malignancy, prolonged use of steroids, rheumatologic disease, liver cirrhosis, renal failure, and septicemia.[5] Among these, previous spine surgery is most common (30%), without regard to the operative technique.[9]

MANAGEMENT

Management can vary according to the type of the causative agent, localization of the disease, neurologic condition, general status of the patient, and stability as well as alignment of the spinal column. The most frequently affected spinal segments are lumbar (58%), thoracic (30%), and cervical (11%).[10] Clinical signs and symptoms caused by spinal infections often are subtle and insidious; therefore, clinical suspicion in patients with nonmechanical pain is important in making a proper diagnosis in early stage of the disease.

Diagnostic studies must be targeted toward anatomic segments of the disease, anatomic localization of the infection, neurologic status of the patient, clinical onset of the disease, the structure of the spine, and the causative agent (Table 1). In many cases, the causative agent is inferred; therefore, the empirical treatment is given. After or even all diagnostic tools are used, biopsy is recommended for the analysis of the organisms.

BIOPSY
Closed (Percutaneous) Biopsy

The rate of definite diagnosis is 68% to 86%.[11–13] Percutaneous CT-guided needle biopsy is found to be safe and its accuracy has been reported up to 70%.[14] Recently, endoscopic biopsy is used in cases of spondylodiscitis, because it also allows discectomy and drainage, and its performance for bacterial recovery is better than CT-guided spinal biopsy.[15,16] The paramedian Kambin triangle for sampling of the intervertebral disc is the primary approach. The Kambin's triangle is defined as a right triangle over the dorsolateral disc. The hypotenuse is the exiting nerve root, the base (width) is the superior border of the caudal vertebra and the height is the dura/traversing nerve root.[17,18] The transpedicular approach is another route that is defined for the percutaneous biopsies.[19,20]

Open Biopsy

Patients who have already received antibiotic therapy can have false-negative biopsy results. If the first biopsy is negative, a second biopsy should be done after an antibiotic-free duration of time. If the second biopsy is also negative, then open surgical biopsy should be considered. Overall,

Table 1
Diagnosis scheme for surgical planning

Anatomic Segments	Anatomic Localization	Neurologic Status	Clinical Onset	Structure of Spine	Causative Agent
Cervical (upper)	Vertebral body	Intact	Acute	Alignment (No/Ne/K)	Pyogenic
Cervical (subaxial)	Intervertebral disc	Neurologic deficit	Subacute	Stability (S or Uns)	Fungal
Thoracic	VB + ID		Chronic	Destruction	Parasitic
Lumbar	Epidural				Others
Sacral	Subdural				
Multisegmental	Intramedullary				
	Paravertebral				

Abbreviations: ID, intervertebral disc; Uns, unstable; K, kyphotic; Ne, neutral; No, normal; S, stable; VB, vertebral body.

30% of biopsies are sterile.[13] Open biopsy is indicated for cases with absolute indications to surgery and negative consecutive biopsy results. It is more accurate, and radical debridement is also possible.

SURGERY

The timing of the surgery is directly related to neurologic status of the patient. Indications for surgery in spinal infections are listed in **Box 1**. A broad range of options for the surgical management of spinal infections that can be chosen according to the pathology, patient status, and structure of the spine include anterior, posterior, combined, and minimally invasive approaches.[10] The choice of the approach is related most closely to the presence of neurologic deficits, the location of the infection, and the degree of associated osseous destruction. The key principles for successful surgical treatment are summarized in **Box 2**.[5] Biomechanical preservation of the spine after infection is crucial for the follow-up period. Before planning the surgery, a thorough evaluation of the spinal stability, alignment, and deformity should be undertaken.

PYOGENIC INFECTIONS
Pyogenic Vertebral Osteomyelitis

Vertebral osteomyelitis and discitis account for 1% to 7% of all bone infections.[5] These bacterial infections often hazard both the integrity of the spinal column and its neural contents. Lumbar lesions

---

Box 1
Indications for surgery in spinal infections

- Biopsy in false-negative biopsy cases
- Neurologic deficit
- Septicemia
- Instability
- Extensive bone destruction
- Deformity
- Intracanal lesion with mass effect
- Unknown etiologies associated with active mass lesion
- Failure of conservative treatment

Data from Duarte RM, Vaccaro AR. Spinal infection: state of the art and management algorithm. Eur Spine J 2013;22(12):2787–99; and Gouliouris T, Aliyu SH, Brown NM. Spondylodiscitis: update on diagnosis and management. J Antimicrob Chemother 2010;65 Suppl 3:iii11–24.

Box 2
The aim of successful surgery

- To diagnose undetermined cases if closed needle biopsy is insufficient;
- To debride the necrotic tissue for increasing the efficiency of the antimicrobial treatment
- To decompress the neural elements and to stabilize the spine in the setting of instability.

Data from Duarte RM, Vaccaro AR. Spinal infection: state of the art and management algorithm. Eur Spine J 2013;22(12):2787–99.

---

with nerve root deficits are usually benign, and the final outcome is satisfactory with and without surgery. However, compression of the thecal sac requires immediate operative intervention. Although upper cervical osteomyelitis is rare, it requires fusion because of the increased risk of instability.

Generally, vertebral bodies and disc spaces are involved in pyogenic vertebral osteomyelitis, so the anterior approach is accepted as the standard method because it provides effective decompression and debridement. Laminectomy is contraindicated in such cases.[3] Radical debridement at the spine comprises resection of the entire infected or necrotic disc and bony tissue, followed by anterior column reconstruction and placement of a strut graft that harvested from iliac bone[3] or titanium cage, as well as a supplemental posterior instrumentation. Fusion is recommended in the appropriate conditions (**Fig. 1**).[21–24] Titanium mesh cages are stated to be as effective as iliac autografts by means of fusion.[25] The metallic implants must be titanium, and not stainless steel, because of bacterial film colonization.[5,24] For 1 level or 2 levels of pyogenic vertebral osteomyelitis, anterior surgery may be enough; however, in cases of long levels, posterior stabilization must be performed.[26] Recent publications demonstrate that anterior fixation after debridement and fusion provides better correction of deformity, shorter operative time, fewer postoperative complications, and earlier rehabilitation than posterior fusion.[25] The intact posterior elements preserve the function of the lumbar spine and improve the quality of life in the postoperative period.[25]

Pyogenic infections rarely affect the posterior elements. Posterior debridement and decompression with laminectomies and posterior fusion should be performed in such cases. Of note, laminectomies should be avoided unless there is a posterior epidural compression and/or infection of the posterior structures. Moreover, to prevent

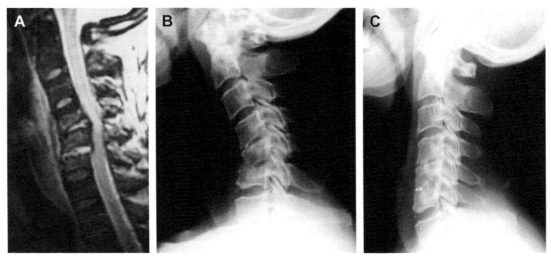

Fig. 1. (A) T2 weighted sagittal MR reveals a severe instability and spinal cord compression that is caused by cervical pyogenic discitis. (B) Preoperative lateral radiogram shows severe kyphosis. (C) Postoperative lateral radiogram demonstrating realignment of the cervical spine after debridement and autogenous bone fusion.

deformity, posterior instrumentation should be performed as far above and below the infected levels as possible; bypassing the infected area may be suitable for some patients during medical therapy.[27] A favorable outcome by controlling the infection and reconstruction of the spinal segment can generally be obtained by medical and/or surgical treatment. Delay in diagnosis and inadequate therapy lead to mortality.

Pyogenic Spondylodiscitis

A needle biopsy sample should be obtained via fluoroscopy, or with CT-guided intervention. Recently endoscopic techniques are used in cases of spondylodiscitis, because they allow discectomy and drainage and their performance for bacterial recovery is better.[15,16,28] Initially conservative treatment with immobilization and antibiotics in cases with minor destruction or minimally invasive abscess reduction, for example, epidural catheters with local antibiotic instillation aiming at a spontaneous fusion of the vertebral bodies or at least fibrous stiffness. However, in some cases, radical surgery with debridement, autologous bone grafting, and stabilization with the possibility to correct deformities is recommended increasingly.[29]

Minimally invasive techniques have had their primary indication in less severe cases with small abscess and little bone destruction. Endoscopic interventions are also appropriate choices for debridement and irrigation, followed by percutaneous drainage.[30] Moreover, percutaneous transpedicular discectomy and drainage are also applicable and result in immediate pain relief.[31]

The posterior approach is indicated in cases of an epidural abscess in the lumbar spine. Large epidural abscesses should be drained emergently because posterior migration of the abscess may result in paraplegia. Patients with multisegmental involvement or distinct substance loss are reported to benefit from a combined approach with ventral debridement and bony bridging, including additional dorsal stabilization.[29]

Pyogenic Epidural Abscess

Most pyogenic epidural abscesses arise from adjacent spondylodiscitis that are often located in the anterior aspect of the spinal canal. Spinal epidural abscesses account for 0.2 to 2 cases per 10,000 hospital admissions.[32] In addition to main surgical indications, epidural abscess even without associated neurologic deficits especially in the cervical and thoracic regions can also be considered as a necessity for operative intervention. Relative indications include uncontrolled pain and contraindications for conservative treatment. Percutaneous endoscopic lavage and drainage are the most recent techniques for diagnostic and therapeutic purposes. This technique is usually the choice for treatment in cases without neurologic deficits and instability. Recent publications have stated that this technique is also effective in multilevel abscesses and recurrent infections.[28] The operative approach depends on the location of the infection. Anterior decompression is necessary for spinal epidural abscess located in the anterior segment of the epidural space; this intervention is usually combined with anterior corpectomy. Laminectomy, hemilaminectomy, or both should be performed for cases that are located posteriorly. Facet joints should be left intact to keep spinal stability and alignment intact after the operation. In children, laminatomy or laminaplasty is preferred because of an attempt to close the posterior covering of the spinal canal is tried after the surgical intervention. After temporary removal of the spinous processes and vertebral laminae, the spinous processes are reconnected to the roots of the vertebral arch of the corresponding vertebrae, once abscess drainage has been undertaken. In most of cases, minimal bone removal without affecting stability is sufficient; therefore, there is no need for additional fusion or stabilization. However, stabilization and fusion should be performed for unstable cases.[22,24] Late diagnosis is associated with mortality.

GRANULOMATOUS INFECTIONS
Tuberculosis

Spinal TB accounts for less than 1% of all TB cases; affected patients are at extremely high risk for neurologic deficits and severe spinal deformities. If the patient is intact neurologically and there is no evidence of spinal instability, treatment should be managed conservatively with chemotherapy and immobilization with a brace or corset.[23,33] Surgical indications are same as for other spinal infections that are summarized in Box 1. Additionally, the presence of kyphosis and instability owing to vertebral corpus destruction may also be considered. Surgical treatment offers an earlier fusion, quicker relief of pain, earlier return to previous activities, less bone loss, and therefore less kyphosis compared with conservative treatment.[23,33,34]

Because the pathology is located typically in the vertebral bodies, debridement should be performed anteriorly. In addition, anterior debridement is essential in cases of neurologic impairment, multilevel involvement, or severe abscess formation. A thorough anterior approach consists of debridement of both the paraspinal abscess and the infected bone; decompression of the spinal canal with tricortical autogenous grafting combined by anterior internal fixation in 1 or 2 level spondylodiscitis should be performed (Figs. 2 and 3). Anterior interbody fusion using a titanium mesh cage also provides solid fusion, maintenance of kyphosis correction, and no recurrence of infection in such patients.[35] Also, it is well-known that infections of the cervical spine require surgical treatment more often when compared with other regions.[36] In the setting of thoracic abscess in at most 2 levels without bony destructions and instability, thoracoscopic drainage is indicated.[37]

Posterior approaches in TB should be the choice of intervention in limited cases that are restricted to posterior elements of the vertebral column and in the setting of a contraindication for anterior internal fixation. Posterior instrumentation and fusion procedures must also be added in cases that were laminectomized. In multilevel (>2 levels) disease, fixed kyphotic deformity, or in cases with a poor quality of adjacent bone strength, staged anterior and posterior intervention is recommended (Fig. 4). Autogenous large fibular or tibial strut grafts are used for larger resection areas. In the setting of greater degrees of kyphotic deformity (>80° of kyphosis) and stiffer curves (25%> flexibility), several types of osteotomies may be helpful in both increasing the curve flexibility and to achieve a successful deformity

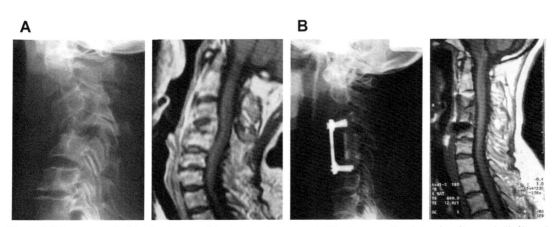

A   **B**

Fig. 2. (A) Severe cervical kyphosis caused by tuberculous spondylitis. Preoperative lateral radiograph (*left*) and sagittal T1 weighted MRI (*right*). (B) The patient underwent an anterior procedure and C4 corpectomy was performed. In addition, an autologous bone graft has been placed and an anterior plate was used for fixation. Postoperative realignment of the C-spine is seen on lateral x-ray (*left*) and sagittal T1 weighted MRI (*right*).

A   B

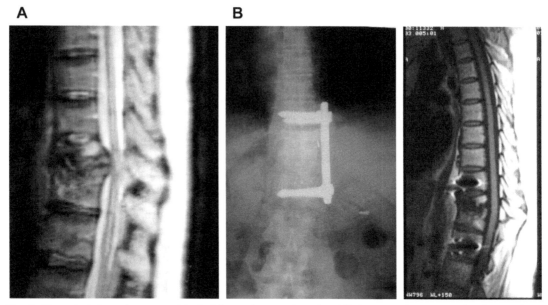

Fig. 3. Thoracic tuberculous spondylodiscitis causing myelopathy. (*A*) Preoperative T2 weighted MRI shows epidural extension with spinal cord compression. (*B*) Postoperative anteroposterior radiograph (*left*) and T1 weighted MRI (*right*) demonstrate instrumentation and relief of the spinal cord.

correction.[38] Being a less adhesive microorganism, *Mycobacterium tuberculosis* produces less ability to adhere the foreign substances, so colonization of metallic implants occurs only rarely. However, the use of stainless steel implants in vertebral osteomyelitis is not recommended.[24,39] The correction of kyphosis should be performed if possible to create normal anatomic degrees, because it allows for more efficient stabilization and early mobilization, and is effective in the maintenance of correction achieved.[35]

Brucellosis

Being the most common zoonosis in endemic areas, brucellosis can account for 21% to 48% of spinal infections.[10] Minority of the cases require surgical intervention. Percutaneous drainage or aspiration of the epidural/paravertebral abscess can be performed instead of surgery.[40] Indications for surgery are same as the other forms of spondylodiscitis.[40,41] For cervical lesions, simple discectomy, discectomy followed by fusion with a

A   B   C   D

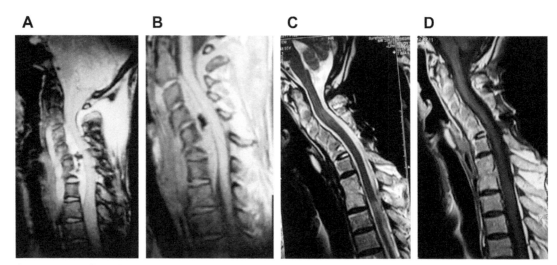

Fig. 4. Severe tuberculosis spondylodiscitis with (*A*) epidural and anterior extension on sagittal T2 weighted and (*B*) contrast-enhanced T1 weighted MRI. After decompression and posterior instrumentation, together with medical treatment, removal of the epidural and soft tissue component with fusion of the vertebral bodies are seen on (*C*) sagittal T2 weighted and (*D*) contrast-enhanced T1 weighted MRI.

tricortical autograft or cage, and corpectomy followed by reconstruction with expandable cage or tricortical autograft with an additional anterior plate should be performed (**Fig. 5**).[42] For the thoracic and lumbar regions, if the disease involves predominantly the anterior elements, anterior debridement plus anterior reconstruction with tricortical autograft or a titanium mesh cage, or anterior debridement plus anterior reconstruction with an additional posterior instrumentation should be implemented.[43] However, in cases limited to the posterior elements without instability, limited laminectomy with debridement is sufficient.[44] Prompt diagnosis and appropriate treatment with antibiotics and surgery—if indicated—is associated with superb prognosis.[40,42]

Actinomycosis

Spinal involvement is unusual and represents less than 5% of the all involved areas.[45] Actinomyosis is usually secondary to an infection of contiguous tissue.[46] The treatment includes antimicrobial therapy with or without surgery. Because the hallmark of infection is the formation of an abscess, to prevent the spread of the disease operative intervention may also be necessary, regardless of the site of infection.[37,45,46] Combined surgical and medical therapy is indicated if the disease becomes complicated. Excellent results are reported with laminectomy and limited debridement when combined with antibiotics.[47]

Nocardiosis

A member of actinomycetes family, *Nocardia* species have been shown as higher aerobic bacteria,

closely related to *Mycobacteria*. Surgery is usually indicated when medical treatment alone has failed, when the disease becomes complicated by an epidural abscess, and in the presence of spinal instability and/or deformity or the existence of progressive neurologic decline.[48] Of the unstable cases, simultaneous spine instrumentation is recommended with wide surgical debridement to living noninfected tissue.[48]

FUNGAL INFECTIONS

Fungal spondylodiscitis is relatively uncommon. *Aspergillus*, *Candida*, and *Cryptococcus* occur worldwide and are known as the most common fungal organisms that invade the spine. Coccidioides and blastomyces are the 2 most common endemic fungi that are responsible from some of the spinal infections.[10,37] Closed needle biopsy is reported to be positive only in up to 50% of affected patients; however, open biopsy is diagnostic in most.[37,49] Targeted pharmacotherapy is the key for success of fungal vertebral osteomyelitis. The objectives of surgical treatment are to diagnose the uncertain issues, decompress the neural tissues, fix the unstable spine, and correct the deformity.[37,49–51] Posterior decompression without fusion should be performed only in the setting of isolated posterior disease without instability.[37,51] Posterior stabilization is required for most patients with posterior element involvement. If there is adequate anterior column support, posterior instrumentation and autograft fusion may provide spinal stability and prevent sagittal plane deformity.[37,51] The anterior approach provides

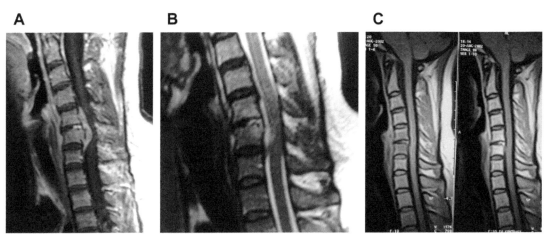

A   **B**   **C**

Fig. 5. (*A*) Cervical discitis and epidural abscess owing to *Brucella* infection with spared vertebral bodies on contrast-enhanced T1 weighted imaging. (*B*) Early postoperative T2 weighted imaging shows that the compression on spinal cord is decreased, but the infection is still continuing. (*C*) Late T1 weighted imaging and contrast-enhanced T1 weighted imaging demonstrate that contrast enhancement of the disc and vertebral bodies consistent with chronic granulomatous infection with disappearance of the epidural component.

the best opportunity for thorough debridement. One other rare fungal spinal infections is mucormycosis.[37,51,52]

PARASITIC INFECTIONS

Parasitic spinal infections are extremely rare. Spinal involvement may occur through either direct hematogenous seeding of the subarachnoid space or inoculation of the attacking organism to the neural structures. A brief description and treatment options for the specific types of common parasitic spinal infections are summarized as follows.

Cysticercosis

The most common parasitic infection affecting the central nervous system, neurocysticercosis is seen endemically. The lesions can be seen in 4 different anatomic locations: extradural, intradural, or subarachnoid spaces (80%) and spinal cord (20%). Owing to the compression of the neural structures, myelopathy and progressive weakness are the most common clinical signs. Surgical excision is necessary to relieve acute and progressive neurologic decline. One must consider arachnoidal scarring and perform sharp dissection, gentle irrigation, and Valsalvas while extirpating such adhesive lesions.[53,54]

Echinococcosis

A worldwide zoonosis, echinococcosis occurs mostly endemically. Being the most common part of bony involvement (45%), spinal disease takes place in only 1% of all hydatid cases. Surgery is the mainstay of the treatment. The cyst should be removed without rupture. Furthermore, the operative field must be irrigated with hypertonic saline solution constantly after removal of the cysts to avoid dissemination. In the setting of multiple involvements, surgery is necessary for segments that are compromised neurologically (Fig. 6). Radical surgical debridement and stabilization of the spine should be performed in vertebral/osseous echinococcosis. To avoid systemic spread and prevent recurrence, adjuvant chemotherapy is crucial. If there is a high risk of cyst rupture, albendazole should be started 4 or more hours before surgery to reach solicidal blood levels.[55–59]

Schistosomiasis

Affecting about 200 million people worldwide, schistosomiasis is seen endemically. Neurosurgical intervention is indicated in the setting of neurologic compromise and/or spinal instability. Decompression, stabilization, and histologic sampling are the goals of surgery.[60–63]

Toxoplasmosis

Although spinal cord disease is uncommon, toxoplasmic infections of the central nervous system are seen usually in patients who are immunocompromised, including those with AIDS or those under immunosuppressive therapy. Neurosurgical intervention is crucial for both histopathologic diagnosis and therapeutic instances in the presence of mass effect and failure of medical therapy. Adjuvant pharmacotherapy should be performed to eradicate the agent.[64,65]

SPINAL INTRADURAL INFECTIONS

Ichor involving the intradural regions is a rare situation both in the modern neurosurgical practice and in antibiotic era. Staphylococcus aureus is

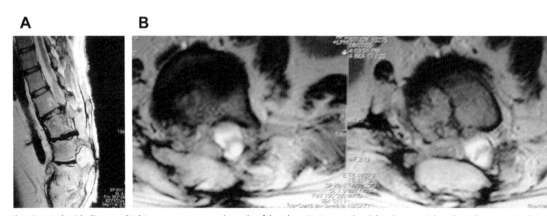

Fig. 6. Hydatid disease (Echinococcus granulosus) of lumbar 3–5 vertebral bodies, epidural and paraspinal soft tissues. (A) Sagittal and (B) axial T2 weighted images show heterogeneous lesions located in the right half of the L3 vertebral body; epidural heterogeneous lesion extending through the right foramina and bony surroundings. Cystic paraspinal soft tissue lesion is also seen.

the most common organism and the thoracolumbar region is the region affected most commonly.[66] In most cases, a secondary cause is also found. Either hematogenous spread or direct inoculation may result as a spinal intradural space infection. The high incidence of morbidity and mortality of such cases may be prevented by early diagnosis and proper treatment. A concise description of the disease is given and treatment strategies of the spinal intradural infections are discussed with respect to the anatomic localization as well as the causative agent.

Spinal Subdural Empyema

The lumbar spine is the most common region for spinal subdural abscesses.[67] In children, the pathogen is mostly TB and located in the thoracic region.[68] Subdural collection especially in cervicothoracic area can cause very rapid deterioration owing to compression of the spinal cord. Therefore, surgical evacuation may be the first choice of the treatment. A posterior approach with laminectomy and duratomy, followed by irrigation, proximally and distally at the site of laminectomy with a rubber catheter, should be the primary choice. This intervention can achieve excellent clinical outcomes.[67]

Spinal Intramedullary Abscess

Because spinal intramedullary abscess is a rare condition, evidence in the literature is limited to case reports. These infections are usually misdiagnosed as tumors and therefore the diagnosis is often late. Surgical excision as limited laminectomies, followed by myelotomies, abscess drainage, and evacuation, should be added to medical therapy if neurologic symptoms progress. Limited laminoplasties with myelotomies and drainage is recommended, especially in children.[69,70] These cases are usually fatal if left undiagnosed and untreated.

Spinal Intradural Fungal Infections

Spinal intradural fungal infections are rare and these are limited to case reports.[71,72] Laminectomy with myelotomy is the treatment of choice.

POSTOPERATIVE SPINAL INFECTIONS

To achieve an accurate diagnosis and successful treatment, the number of techniques and invasive procedures continue to increase in the area of spinal surgery. The incidence of surgical site infection after discectomy, decompressive laminectomy, and fusion is as high as approximately 3%; however, it increases to as great as

12% with the addition of instrumentation.[24,73] Moreover, instrumented cases require a longer duration of antibiotic therapy, more debridement surgeries, and have had a higher rate of treatment failure.[74] Postoperative spinal infections are either located in the skin and/or subcutaneous tissue (superficial infections) or below the muscle fascia (deep infections). These infections can be seen either as alone or in combination as discitis, spondylodiscitis, epidural abscesses, and surgical wound infections.[49,75] Risk factors are summarized in **Box 3**.[76]

Successful infection management begins preoperatively with aseptic technique and proper antibiotic prophylaxis administration. Up to a 60% reduction in the incidence of surgical site infections can be achieved with prophylactic antibiotics applied 60 minutes before a procedure. In the presence of prolonged procedures with gross contamination and significant blood loss (>1 L), an additional dose of antibiotics should be administered.[24,73]

Spinal Instrumentation and Infection

Up to 11.9% of patients who undergo spinal surgery with instrumentation may develop an infection, depending on the diagnosis and complexity of the initial operative procedure. Beside appropriate use of antimicrobial agents, initial debridement with implant retention is usually performed for both goals, resulting in implant retention rates of 40% to 100%.[77] Implant retention may prevent bacterial eradication because of the presence of

---

Box 3
Risk factors for postoperative spine infections

Preoperative

Older age

Obesity

Smoking

Previous infection

Diabetes

Postoperative

Revision surgery

Use of instrumentation

Increased intraoperative blood loss

Prolonged operative time[79]

Data from Smith JS, Shaffrey CI, Sansur CA, et al. Rates of infection after spine surgery based on 108,419 procedures: a report from the Scoliosis Research Society Morbidity and Mortality Committee. Spine (Phila Pa 1976) 2011;36(7):556–63.

biofilm on metal hardware, which diminishes the effect of antibiotics.[78] Some authors claim that, when the infected instruments are retained in the body, and despite aggressive antibiotic treatment, histologic evidence of an active infection remains and the colonization of bacteria continues, so evidence of subclinical infection occurs.[79,80] In other words, the bacteria stand as a biofilm phenotype on the avascular implant surface and behave as a barrier to the both host immune response and antibiotic therapy.[75] Yet, if the hardware is removed before fusion as an attempt to control the infection, this may result in spinal instability, causing clinical symptoms of back pain, radicular pain, and neurologic deficits.[77] Curve progression after removal of posterior instrumentation remains a concern. Muschik and colleagues[81] demonstrated that curve progression after implant removal for infection has been significant if reinstrumentation has not taken place. In the presence of superficial infection, short fusion (<3 levels), cervical spine surgery, methicillin-sensitive S aureus infection, and no evidence of fusion are predictors of early resolution and they can be often treated while retaining implants. However, in the setting of late infection, long instrumented fusions (>6 levels), polymicrobial infections, and Propionibacterium acnes infections, conservative approach generally fails. In early infections, debridement with implant retention is ideal and should be attempted. Rates of successful implant retention of 92% to 100% have been reported by authors who have used multiple debridements in combination with continuous irrigation, antibiotic-impregnated cement beads, or secondary wound closure.[82,83] Hardware removal after multiple debridement is sometimes required. If fusion is not complete at the time of removal, however, debate is ongoing about whether reimplantation should be performed above and below the infected area with titanium implants, because they are less adherent to the bacterial glycocalyx.[27,75] In late infections—those occurring several months or years after the initial operation—implant removal is preferable because of the documented bony fusion or difficulty in resolving the infection. However, these patients must closely be followed because of the increased risk of pseudoarthrosis.[82]

Postoperative Discitis

The reported incidence for postoperative infection of the disc space has been estimated as 0.2% to 3% of all lumbar discectomies.[82,84] Low back pain is the common complaint, and sometimes can lead to a diagnosis delay because of its insidious onset and uncertain course.[82,84] The organism located on the patient's skin can produce an iatrogenic spondylodiscitis if incomplete asepsis is done. Needle biopsy is preferred to an open intervention. Of note, although it is more invasive, open biopsy is more likely to isolate the causative agent. Antibiotic therapy should be adjusted based on the infectious agents and their sensitivity to antibiotics those reported on antibiograms.[84] Surgery should be reserved for progression of disease on MRI despite proper antibiotic therapy, neurologic deterioration owing to the involvement of spinal canal, and/or vertebral body destruction causing deformity. In early postoperative discitis with minimal vertebral body involvement, debridement by percutaneous or endoscopic techniques is reported to be sufficent.[30,82] Depending on the localization of the infection, anterior only or posterior only careful reexploration and debridement may be sufficient. Autologous bone graft as an interbody spacer is also recommended by some authors to minimize the risk of recurrent infection.[82] Stabilization and fusion should be done in the setting of instability (Fig. 7). The overall prognosis is good with all patients returning to work without any long-term disability.

Postoperative Epidural Abscess

Because it involves the potential for neurologic destruction, prompt diagnosis and treatment of postoperative epidural abscess is crucial. Diagnosis may be difficult in the early postoperative period. Increased back pain, systemic symptoms owing to infection, and an eventual neurologic deficit may be seen with progression of the disease. Epidural abscesses can be managed conservatively when small. Immediate surgical decompression and drainage is the treatment of choice if small collections continue to progress despite antibiotic therapy and/or in the setting of neurologic deficits.[75,82] The surgical approach depends on the location of the abscess as well as the extent of involvement. Posteriorly located abscesses are usually treated with a posterior decompression, such as a laminectomy. Because of the anteriorly seated granulation tissue that arises from discitis and/or osteomyelitis, anterior surgery is recommended in the presence of anterior disease.[75] Early recognition and rapid intervention are 2 major prognostic factors for a favorable outcome.[75]

Postoperative Wound Infection

Wound closure should be performed primarily or with a vacuum dressing. However, a wound may be left open if indicated.[24] A muscle flap may be required in the setting of large soft tissue defects.[82]

A   B   C

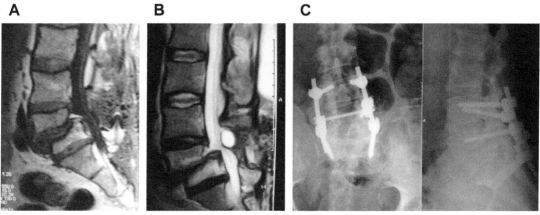

Fig. 7. Late complication of postoperative pyogenic discitis. Sagittal T1 weighted image (A) and T2 weighted image (B) reveal severe deformity with anterolisthesis. Postoperative (C) anteroposterior (left) and lateral (right) radiographs show realignment and healing after decompression and fusion.

Postoperative Infections After Percutaneous Procedures

Minimally invasive techniques have lower infection rates than open surgery.[85] Most of the published cases have had multiple comorbidities or immunosuppression that allow low-virulence organisms to grow and multiply at the operation site.[86] The mainstay of treatment is surgical debridement and stabilization after unsuccessful conservative treatment. There are some cases reported in literature from laminectomy only to anterior and posterior stabilization simultaneously. Conservative treatment has been preferred in some very severe ill cases with intravenous antibiotics.[85–87]

PEARLS, PITFALLS, AND NORMAL VARIANTS

Pearls
1. Severe neurologic deficit, epidural abscess, deformity, and instability are the main indications for surgical treatment in spine infections.
2. Risk factors for spine infection after spine surgery are mostly related to preoperative condition of the patient and perioperative handling.
3. Defining the anatomic location of the infection (anterior vs posterior column) is the key point in planning the surgical approach.

Pitfalls
1. Misdiagnosis of intramedullary abscess as intramedullary tumor.
2. Performing laminectomy in severe anterior column deformity and destruction.
3. Performing surgery in fungal infection without a microscope.
4. Conservative treatment in epidural abscess collection with neurologic deficits.

5. Not to consider specific and nonspecific spondylodiscitis as a differential diagnostic parameter while evaluating chronic low back pain.

WHAT THE REFERRING PHYSICIAN NEEDS TO KNOW

Is this an emergent case?
Is there any spinal cord compression?
Is there any spinal column instability?

FUTURE CONSIDERATIONS AND SUMMARY

Appropriate timing and planning of an operative procedure combined with adequate medical therapy may improve the prognosis. With the advent of antibiotics, improved techniques of management, and early recognition, mortality associated with spinal infections has decreased significantly.[5] A favorable outcome by controlling the infection and reconstruction of the spinal segment can generally be obtained by medical and/or surgical treatment. Delay in diagnosis and inadequate therapy leads to mortality. Severe neurologic deficit, epidural abscess, deformity, and instability are the main indications for surgical treatment in spine infections. The appropriate surgical techniques are:

a. Percutaneous or endoscopic biopsy plus medical treatment plus external immobilization and bed rest.
b. Minimally invasive debridement of the infection via endoscopy or epidural catheter and external immobilization and bed rest.
c. Anterior approach
d. Posterior approach
e. Combined

REFERENCES

1. Krodel A, Sturz H. Differentiated surgical and conservative treatment of spondylitis and spondylodiscitis. Z Orthop Ihre Grenzgeb 1989;127(5):587–96.

2. Mintz CJ, Benson DR. Pyogenic vertebral osteomyelitis in the lumbosacral junction. In: Marquillies YJ, Flomann Y, Farcy JP, et al, editors. Lumbosacral and spinopelvic fixation. 1st edition. Philadelphia: Lippincott-Raven; 1996. p. 93–104.

3. Ruf M, Stoltze D, Merk HR, et al. Treatment of vertebral osteomyelitis by radical debridement and stabilization using titanium mesh cages. Spine (Phila Pa 1976) 2007;32(9):E275–80.

4. Sobottke R, Seifert H, Fatkenheuer G, et al. Current diagnosis and treatment of spondylodiscitis. Dtsch Arztebl Int 2008;105(10):181–7.

5. Duarte RM, Vaccaro AR. Spinal infection: state of the art and management algorithm. Eur Spine J 2013; 22(12):2787–99.

6. Grammatico L, Baron S, Rusch E, et al. Epidemiology of vertebral osteomyelitis (VO) in France: analysis of hospital-discharge data 2002–2003. Epidemiol Infect 2008;136(5):653–60.

7. Hadjipavlou AG, Mader JT, Necessary JT, et al. Hematogenous pyogenic spinal infections and their surgical management. Spine (Phila Pa 1976) 2000; 25(13):1668–79.

8. Turunc T, Demiroglu YZ, Uncu H, et al. A comparative analysis of tuberculous, brucellar and pyogenic spontaneous spondylodiscitis patients. J Infect 2007;55(2):158–63.

9. Kasliwal MK, Tan LA, Traynelis VC. Infection with spinal instrumentation: Review of pathogenesis, diagnosis, prevention, and management. Surg Neurol Int 2013;4(Suppl 5):S392–403.

10. Gouliouris T, Aliyu SH, Brown NM. Spondylodiscitis: update on diagnosis and management. J Antimicrob Chemother 2010;65(Suppl 3):iii11–24.

11. Armstrong P, Chalmers AH, Green G, et al. Needle aspiration/biopsy of the spine in suspected disc infection. Br J Radiol 1978;51(605):333–7.

12. Ottolenghi CE, Schajowicz F, Deschant FA. Aspiration biopsy of the cervical spine. Technique and results in thirty-four cases. J Bone Joint Surg Am 1964; 46:715–33.

13. Sapico FL, Montgomerie JZ. Pyogenic vertebral osteomyelitis: report of nine cases and review of the literature. Rev Infect Dis 1979;1(5):754–76.

14. Gasbarrini A, Boriani L, Salvadori C, et al. Biopsy for suspected spondylodiscitis. Eur Rev Med Pharmacol Sci 2012;16(Suppl 2):26–34.

15. Guerado E, Cervan AM. Surgical treatment of spondylodiscitis. An update. Int Orthop 2012;36(2): 413–20.

16. Yang SC, Fu TS, Chen LH, et al. Identifying pathogens of spondylodiscitis: percutaneous endoscopy or CT-guided biopsy. Clin Orthop Relat Res 2008; 466(12):3086–92.

17. Xin G, Shi-Sheng H, Hai-Long Z. Morphometric analysis of the YESS and TESSYS techniques of percutaneous transforaminal endoscopic lumbar discectomy. Clin Anat 2013;26(6):728–34.

18. Kambin P, Sampson S. Posterolateral percutaneous suction-excision of herniated lumbar intervertebral discs. Report of interim results. Clin Orthop Relat Res 1986;(207):37–43.

19. Renfrew DL, Whitten CG, Wiese JA, et al. CT-guided percutaneous transpedicular biopsy of the spine. Radiology 1991;180(2):574–6.

20. Hadjipavlou AG, Crow WN, Borowski A, et al. Percutaneous transpedicular discectomy and drainage in pyogenic spondylodiscitis. Am J Orthop (Belle Mead NJ) 1998;27(3):188–97.

21. Robinson Y, Tschoeke SK, Kayser R, et al. Reconstruction of large defects in vertebral osteomyelitis with expandable titanium cages. Int Orthop 2009; 33(3):745–9.

22. Aho C, Wang MY. Pyogenic infections of the spine. In: Anderson DG, Vaccaro AR, editors. Decision making in spinal care. New York: Thieme; 2007. p. 338–43.

23. An HS. Spinal infections. In: An HS, editor. Synopsis of spine surgery. 1st edition. Baltimore (MD): Williams & Wilkins; 1998. p. 319–27.

24. Long WD III, Whang PG. Infection. In: Baaj AA, Mummaneni PV, Uribe JS, et al, editors. Handbook of spine surgery. 1st edition. New York: Thieme; 2012. p. 127–35.

25. Si M, Yang ZP, Li ZF, et al. Anterior versus posterior fixation for the treatment of lumbar pyogenic vertebral osteomyelitis. Orthopedics 2013;36(6):831–6.

26. Hee HT, Majd ME, Holt RT, et al. Better treatment of vertebral osteomyelitis using posterior stabilization and titanium mesh cages. J Spinal Disord Tech 2002;15(2):149–56 [discussion: 156].

27. Mohamed AS, Yoo J, Hart R, et al. Posterior fixation without debridement for vertebral body osteomyelitis and discitis. Neurosurg Focus 2014;37(2):E6.

28. Yang SC, Chen WJ, Chen HS, et al. Extended indications of percutaneous endoscopic lavage and drainage for the treatment of lumbar infectious spondylitis. Eur Spine J 2014;23(4):846–53.

29. Heyde CE, Boehm H, El Saghir H, et al. Surgical treatment of spondylodiscitis in the cervical spine: a minimum 2-year follow-up. Eur Spine J 2006; 15(9):1380–7.

30. Ito M, Abumi K, Kotani Y, et al. Clinical outcome of posterolateral endoscopic surgery for pyogenic spondylodiscitis: results of 15 patients with serious comorbid conditions. Spine (Phila Pa 1976) 2007; 32(2):200–6.

31. Hadjipavlou AG, Katonis PK, Gaitanis IN, et al. Percutaneous transpedicular discectomy and

drainage in pyogenic spondylodiscitis. Eur Spine J 2004;13(8):707–13.

32. Mackenzie AR, Laing RB, Smith CC, et al. Spinal epidural abscess: the importance of early diagnosis and treatment. J Neurol Neurosurg Psychiatr 1998; 65(2):209–12.

33. Peppers TA. Atypical infections of the spine: tuberculosis and fungal infections. In: Anderson DG, Vaccaro AR, editors. Decision making in spinal care. New York: Thieme; 2007. p. 345–50.

34. Garg RK, Somvanshi DS. Spinal tuberculosis: a review. J Spinal Cord Med 2011;34(5):440–54.

35. Erturer E, Tezer M, Aydogan M, et al. The results of simultaneous posterior-anterior-posterior surgery in multilevel tuberculosis spondylitis associated with severe kyphosis. Eur Spine J 2010;19(12):2209–15.

36. Schinkel C, Gottwald M, Andress HJ. Surgical treatment of spondylodiscitis. Surg Infect (Larchmt) 2003;4(4):387–91.

37. Kim CW, Currier BL, Eismont FJ. Infections of the spine. In: Herkowitz HN, Garfin SR, Eismont FJ, et al, editors. Rothman-simeone the spine. 6th edition. Philadelphia: Elsevier-Saunders; 2011. p. 1513–70.

38. Issack PS, Boachie-Adjei O. Surgical correction of kyphotic deformity in spinal tuberculosis. Int Orthop 2012;36(2):353–7.

39. Oga M, Arizono T, Takasita M, et al. Evaluation of the risk of instrumentation as a foreign body in spinal tuberculosis. Clinical and biologic study. Spine (Phila Pa 1976) 1993;18(13):1890–4.

40. Alp E, Doganay M. Current therapeutic strategy in spinal brucellosis. Int J Infect Dis 2008;12(6): 573–7.

41. Ulu-Kilic A, Karakas A, Erdem H, et al. Update on treatment options for spinal brucellosis. Clin Microbiol Infect 2014;20(2):O75–82.

42. Ekici MA, Ozbek Z, Gokoglu A, et al. Surgical management of cervical spinal epidural abscess caused by Brucella melitensis: report of two cases and review of the literature. J Korean Neurosurg Soc 2012;51(6):383–7.

43. Ozalay M, Sahin O, Derincek A, et al. Non-tuberculous thoracic and lumbar spondylodiscitis: single-stage anterior debridement and reconstruction, combined with posterior instrumentation and grafting. Acta Orthop Belg 2010;76(1):100–6.

44. Daglioglu E, Bayazit N, Okay O, et al. Lumbar epidural abscess caused by Brucella species: report of two cases. Neurocirugia (Astur) 2009; 20(2):159–62.

45. Duvignaud A, Ribeiro E, Moynet D, et al. Cervical spondylitis and spinal abscess due to Actinomyces meyeri. Braz J Infect Dis 2014;18(1):106–9.

46. Honda H, Bankowski MJ, Kajioka EH, et al. Thoracic vertebral actinomycosis: Actinomyces israelii and Fusobacterium nucleatum. J Clin Microbiol 2008; 46(6):2009–14.

47. Yung BC, Cheng JC, Chan TT, et al. Aggressive thoracic actinomycosis complicated by vertebral osteomyelitis and epidural abscess leading to spinal cord compression. Spine (Phila Pa 1976) 2000; 25(6):745–8.

48. Graat HC, Van Ooij A, Day GA, et al. Nocardia farcinica spinal osteomyelitis. Spine (Phila Pa 1976) 2002;27(10):E253–7.

49. Rowshan K, Eismont FJ. Spine infections. In: Rao RD, editor. Orthopaedic knowledge update: spine 4. 4th edition. Rosemont (IL): American Academy of Orthopaedic Surgeons; 2012. p. 525–34.

50. Zussman BM, Penn DL, Harrop JS. Surgical management of fungal vertebral osteomyelitis. JHN Journal 2011;6(2):6–10.

51. Kim CW, Perry A, Currier B, et al. Fungal infections of the spine. Clin Orthop Relat Res 2006;444:92–9.

52. Chen F, Lu G, Kang Y, et al. Mucormycosis spondylodiscitis after lumbar disc puncture. Eur Spine J 2006;15(3):370–6.

53. Alsina GA, Johnson JP, McBride DQ, et al. Spinal neurocysticercosis. Neurosurg Focus 2002;12(6):e8.

54. Shin SH, Hwang BW, Lee SJ, et al. Primary extensive spinal subarachnoid cysticercosis. Spine (Phila Pa 1976) 2012;37(19):E1221–4.

55. Steinmetz S, Racloz G, Stern R, et al. Treatment challenges associated with bone echinococcosis. J Antimicrob Chemother 2014;69(3):821–6.

56. Pamir MN, Ozduman K, Elmaci I. Spinal hydatid disease. Spinal Cord 2002;40(4):153–60.

57. Neumayr A, Tamarozzi F, Goblirsch S, et al. Spinal cystic echinococcosis–a systematic analysis and review of the literature: part 2. Treatment, follow-up and outcome. PLoS Negl Trop Dis 2013;7(9):e2458.

58. Neumayr A, Tamarozzi F, Goblirsch S, et al. Spinal cystic echinococcosis–a systematic analysis and review of the literature: part 1. Epidemiology and anatomy. PLoS Negl Trop Dis 2013;7(9):e2450.

59. Lotfinia I, Sayyahmelli S, Mahdkhah A, et al. Intradural extramedullary primary hydatid cyst of the spine: a case report and review of literature. Eur Spine J 2013;22(Suppl 3):S329–36.

60. Salim AD, Arbab MA, El Hassan LA, et al. Schistosomiasis of the spinal cord: report of 5 cases from Sudan. East Mediterr Health J 2012;18(3):294–7.

61. Kamel MH, Murphy M, Kelleher M, et al. Schistosomiasis of the spinal cord presenting as progressive myelopathy. Case report. J Neurosurg Spine 2005; 3(1):61–3.

62. Gryseels B, Polman K, Clerinx J, et al. Human schistosomiasis. Lancet 2006;368(9541):1106–18.

63. Go JL, Rothman S, Prosper A, et al. Spine infections. Neuroimaging Clin N Am 2012;22(4):755–72.

64. Cosan TE, Kabukcuoglu S, Arslantas A, et al. Spinal toxoplasmic arachnoiditis associated with osteoid formation: a rare presentation of toxoplasmosis. Spine (Phila Pa 1976) 2001;26(15):1726–8.

65. Garcia-Gubern C, Fuentes CR, Colon-Rolon L, et al. Spinal cord toxoplasmosis as an unusual presentation of AIDS: case report and review of the literature. Int J Emerg Med 2010;3(4):439–42.

66. Khalil JG, Nassr A, Diehn FE, et al. Thoracolumbosacral spinal subdural abscess: magnetic resonance imaging appearance and limited surgical management. Spine (Phila Pa 1976) 2013;38(13): E844–7.

67. Lim HY, Choi HJ, Kim S, et al. Chronic spinal subdural abscess mimicking an intradural-extramedullary tumor. Eur Spine J 2013;22(Suppl 3):S497–500.

68. Sandler AL, Thompson D, Goodrich JT, et al. Infections of the spinal subdural space in children: a series of 11 contemporary cases and review of all published reports. A multinational collaborative effort. Childs Nerv Syst 2013;29(1):105–17.

69. Sinha P, Parekh T, Pal D. Intramedullary abscess of the upper cervical spinal cord. Unusual presentation and dilemmas of management: case report. Clin Neurol Neurosurg 2013;115(9):1845–50.

70. Mohindra S, Sodhi HS, Aggarwal A. Management problems of intramedullary holocord abscess: an illustration in a pediatric case. Childs Nerv Syst 2012;28(4):637–40.

71. Saigal G, Donovan Post MJ, Kozic D. Thoracic intradural Aspergillus abscess formation following epidural steroid injection. AJNR Am J Neuroradiol 2004;25(4):642–4.

72. Hott JS, Horn E, Sonntag VK, et al. Intramedullary histoplasmosis spinal cord abscess in a nonendemic region: case report and review of the literature. J Spinal Disord Tech 2003;16(2):212–5.

73. Chaudhary SB, Vives MJ, Basra SK, et al. Postoperative spinal wound infections and postprocedural diskitis. J Spinal Cord Med 2007;30(5):441–51.

74. Pull ter Gunne AF, Cohen DB. Incidence, prevalence, and analysis of risk factors for surgical site infection following adult spinal surgery. Spine (Phila Pa 1976) 2009;34(13):1422–8.

75. Nasto LA, Colangelo D, Rossi B, et al. Post-operative spondylodiscitis. Eur Rev Med Pharmacol Sci 2012;16(Suppl 2):50–7.

76. Smith JS, Shaffrey CI, Sansur CA, et al. Rates of infection after spine surgery based on 108,419 procedures: a report from the Scoliosis Research Society Morbidity and Mortality Committee. Spine (Phila Pa 1976) 2011;36(7):556–63.

77. Ishii M, Iwasaki M, Ohwada T, et al. Postoperative deep surgical-site infection after instrumented spinal surgery: a multicenter study. Global Spine J 2013; 3(2):95–102.

78. Costerton JW. Biofilm theory can guide the treatment of device-related orthopaedic infections. Clin Orthop Relat Res 2005;(437):7–11.

79. Sampedro MF, Huddleston PM, Piper KE, et al. A biofilm approach to detect bacteria on removed spinal implants. Spine (Phila Pa 1976) 2010;35(12): 1218–24.

80. Ochoa G. Infections of the spine. In: Aebi M, Arlet V, Webb JK, editors. AO Spine manual. New York: Thieme; 2007. p. 257–99.

81. Muschik M, Luck W, Schlenzka D. Implant removal for late-developing infection after instrumented posterior spinal fusion for scoliosis: reinstrumentation reduces loss of correction. A retrospective analysis of 45 cases. Eur Spine J 2004;13(7):645–51.

82. Hegde V, Meredith DS, Kepler CK, et al. Management of postoperative spinal infections. World J Orthop 2012;3(11):182–9.

83. Bible JE, Biswas D, Devin CJ. Postoperative infections of the spine. Am J Orthop (Belle Mead NJ) 2011;40(12):E264–71.

84. Adam D, Papacocea T, Hornea I, et al. Postoperative spondylodiscitis. A review of 24 consecutive patients. Chirurgia (Bucur) 2014;109(1):90–4.

85. Uribe JS, Deukmedjian AR, Mummaneni PV, et al. Complications in adult spinal deformity surgery: an analysis of minimally invasive, hybrid, and open surgical techniques. Neurosurg Focus 2014;36(5): E15.

86. Abdelrahman H, Siam AE, Shawky A, et al. Infection after vertebroplasty or kyphoplasty. A series of nine cases and review of literature. Spine J 2013;13(12): 1809–17.

87. Anand N, Baron EM, Khandehroo B, et al. Long-term 2- to 5-year clinical and functional outcomes of minimally invasive surgery for adult scoliosis. Spine (Phila Pa 1976) 2013;38(18):1566–75.

Overview of the Complications and Sequelae in Spinal Infections

 CrossMark

Jef Huyskens, MD*, Johan Van Goethem, MD, PhD*,
Marguerite Faure, MD, Luc van den Hauwe, MD,
Frank De Belder, MD, Caroline Venstermans, MD,
Paul M. Parizel, MD, PhD

KEYWORDS

• Spondylitis • Discitis • Spondylodiscitis • MR imaging

KEY POINTS

- Worldwide most complications of spondylitis are still seen in cases of tuberculous spondylitis.
- However, in Western countries more and more complications are seen in postoperative spondylitis.
- The number of immunosuppressed patients is rising. They are more susceptible to infections in general and spinal infections in particular.
- Clinicians need to be aware of the possible slow progressive course with relatively little and nonspecific symptoms of spinal infectious disease.
- Early diagnosis depends mainly on biochemical and imaging findings. With the advent of MR imaging patients are diagnosed earlier and hence can be treated conservatively.
- Progressive disease with spinal instability is generally treated as spinal trauma.

INTRODUCTION

Spondylitis, or infection of the spine (from Ancient Greek σπόνδυλος [spóndulos] = spine), is a spectrum of diseases involving the bone, disks, and/or ligaments.[1,2] Therefore, in this spectrum we include spondylitis (also infection of the vertebral body), discitis, spondylodiscitis, vertebral osteomyelitis, pyogenic facet arthritis, epidural infections, meningitis, polyradiculitis, and myelitis.

This article mainly discusses discitis, spondylitis, and spondylodiscitis, primarily because these occur most frequently. Osteomyelitis of the posterior elements is rare and should raise suspicion of tuberculosis or an iatrogenic cause.[1,2]

Mostly spondylitis and discitis are caused by hematogenous spread of an infection located elsewhere in the body. Only rarely is it nonhematogenous and in these cases it is mostly iatrogenic, caused by interventional procedures, surgical intervention, penetrating trauma, contiguous infection, or direct inoculation.[1–5]

In ancient history the most common cause of spinal infection was *Mycobacterium tuberculosis*.[2,5] In most Western countries this is not endemic. However, the incidence of tuberculosis is rising, especially in immunocompromised patients.[2] The most frequent cause in western countries is the pyogenic form of spondylodiscitis, most commonly by *Staphylococcus aureus* infection (60%).[1–5]

Spinal infections are most frequently located at the lumbar level (60%), less frequently at the thoracic level (30%), and only in 10% at the cervical level. Only rarely is it located in the sacrum.[4]

Disclosures: None.
Department of Radiology, Antwerp University Hospital, University of Antwerp, Wilrijkstraat 10, Edegem 2650, Belgium
* Corresponding authors.
E-mail addresses: jef_huyskens@hotmail.com; johan.vangoethem@uantwerpen.be

Neuroimag Clin N Am 25 (2015) 309–321
http://dx.doi.org/10.1016/j.nic.2015.01.007
1052-5149/15/$ – see front matter © 2015 Elsevier Inc. All rights reserved.

There is a difference in spondylitis in children versus adults. Until the age of 15 years, children have numerous paravertebral and intraosseous collateral arteries and a direct blood supply to the intervertebral disks, reaching the nucleus pulposus, and thus the infection is primarily discogenic. The course of discitis in children is often benign and is treated with antibiotics. Surgical abscesses are rare and drainage or decompression is hardly ever needed.[1–5] This blood supply regresses in adults and predominantly the end-artery metaphyseal branches remain. The infection usually begins in the anterior subchondral regions and spreads secondarily to the disk.[1–6]

MR imaging is the modality of choice in the evaluation and diagnosis of spinal infections in an early stage.[7–9] It is often not helpful for routine follow-up of the disease because it does not correlate with the clinical course. It sometimes shows disease progression despite treatment.[2,4]

Computed tomography is sensitive for delineating bone and evaluating bone destruction, but also allows imaging a larger field of view, which can be useful in case of extensive extravertebral expansion, such as in the abdomen, chest, or mediastinum.[2,4,5]

Radiographs usually remain normal 2 to 8 weeks after the onset of infection but are still useful for the evaluation of spinal alignment. Therefore, plain radiographs often serve as a baseline investigation for further follow-up.[1,2,4,5]

Bone scintigraphy shows arterial hyperemia and a progressive focal uptake and is therefore highly sensitive.[1,2,4,5,7] Tuberculosis infections, however, are cold in 35% to 40% of cases.

On PET scan spinal infections are usually fluorodeoxyglucose avid.[4] Therefore, nuclear medicine is used in the work-up of spondylodiscitis in combination with MR imaging. Spinal infections can be an incidental finding on nuclear imaging studies, necessitating further work-up.

Mortality rates vary between 2% and 11% and are remarkably better than before the use of effective antibiotics pre–World War II, with a mortality rate of about 70%.[3–5] The most common complication of spondylitis is abscess formation in the psoas muscle. Epidural abscesses and compression fractures are not uncommon. Mechanical compression, however, is the most common cause of functional compromise of the spinal cord. Ischemic compromise of the spinal cord is infrequent.[1–4,6] Extensive destruction of the vertebral spine is frequently seen in endemic areas of *M tuberculosis* and commonly is not encountered in the Western world.[1–4]

SEQUELAE OF POSTOPERATIVE INFECTIONS

The postoperative spine is discussed separately, because symptoms, clinical presentation, and complications may differ widely. Postoperative spondylodiscitis occurs in 0.1% to 4% of all spinal procedures, depending on the literature. It commonly occurs 1 to 4 weeks after surgery, chemonucleolysis, and even diagnostic interventional procedures and accounts for 20% to 30% of all cases of spondylodiscitis.[4,6] It typically presents with severe back pain, with or without radiculopathy.[4,6]

It is a serious complication and may lead to significant morbidity and even mortality. It can result in bacteremia and septicemia; the need for removal of implants, and loosening of the material or subsidence of cages; and pseudoarthrosis. In time it can cause instability.

Early diagnosis and treatment are important to shorten the disease course and therefore reduce the sequelae. Although the incidence of postoperative infections is decreasing because of better technical and prophylactic measures, it has not been completely eliminated.[5]

The infection is mostly caused by intraoperative contamination, although a preoperative or perioperative infection at another site or an underlying immunocompromising condition can also predispose. The organisms involved are usually *Staphylococcus epidermidis* or *S aureus*.[2,4,5]

Diagnosing spondylodiscitis with the help of MR imaging is typically a challenging problem in the postoperative spine. The operated disk level always shows changes caused by the surgical intervention and the accompanying postoperative inflammatory response. Bone marrow edema in the adjacent end plates is commonly seen in postoperative patients even when not infected. In addition, normal contrast enhancement caused by fibrosis can be seen in the disk and along the end plates postoperatively (**Figs. 1** and **2**). MR imaging is the only imaging modality for the diagnosis of postoperative spondylodiscitis.[1,7–9]

EXTRASPINAL SPREAD OF INFECTION

If spondylitis or in rare occasions septic facet arthritis is left untreated it can directly spread to the surrounding tissues. This could result in phlegmon or abscess formation in the surrounding soft tissues and even in the epidural space (see **Fig. 2**). In general epidural involvement is reported in 32% of the cases.[1,2,4,5,10]

A phlegmon is the inflammation caused by tissue infiltration. Abscess formation with necrosis,

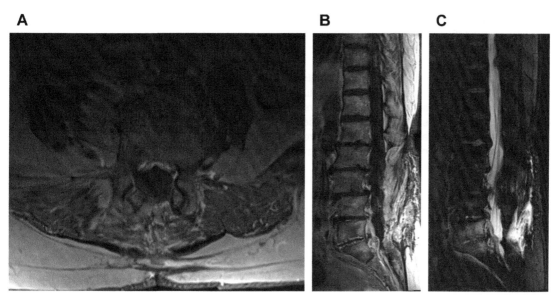

Fig. 1. Patient 1, a 66-year-old woman with progressive immobilizing radicular back pain. MR imaging (A) axial contrast-enhanced (CE) T1, (B) sagittal CE T1, (C) sagittal short TI inversion recovery (STIR). After broad laminectomy there is a spondylodiscitis of L5-S1 with phlegmon formation in the anterior epidural space with a so-called curtain sign on the axial CE T1.

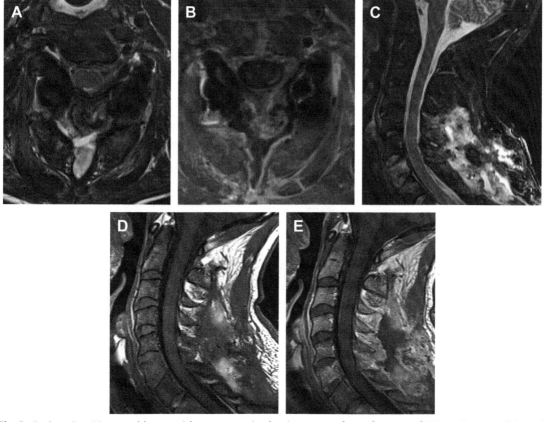

Fig. 2. Patient 2, a 38-year-old man with postoperative laminectomy after a fracture of C6. MR imaging (A) axial T2, (B) axial CE T1, (C) sagittal STIR, (D) sagittal T1, (E) sagittal CE T1. Spondylitis of C6 postlaminectomy, abscess in the posterior elements with expansion in the epidural space.

however, is a collection of pus. It is differentiated by T1-weighted MR imaging with intravenous gadolinium, because a phlegmon is an inhomogeneous enhancing soft tissue mass and an abscess presents as a thick rim-enhancing collection.[2,4,10] This is an important difference because of the poorer prognosis of an abscess versus epidural granulation tissue.[4] Mostly an abscess needs surgical or percutaneous drainage, whereas a phlegmon is treated conservatively with intravenous antibiotics (Figs. 3 and 4).

Some authors even associate an abscess with acute disease and granulation tissue with a chronic one. There is nevertheless no real distinction,

making it more a continuum of the same infectious process.[10] We use both terms.

The most common findings in spondylitis are psoas phlegmons and abscesses (Fig. 5). They are mostly treated with intravenous antibiotics and in more severe therapy-resistant cases with percutaneous drainage. According to the literature 90% of the cervical, 33% of the thoracic, and 24% of the lumbar located spondylodiscitis develop an epidural abscess (see Fig. 4).[4]

Infectious pyogenic spondylitis can digest disks and end plates by proteolytic enzymes, produced by pyogenic organisms, most commonly S aureus

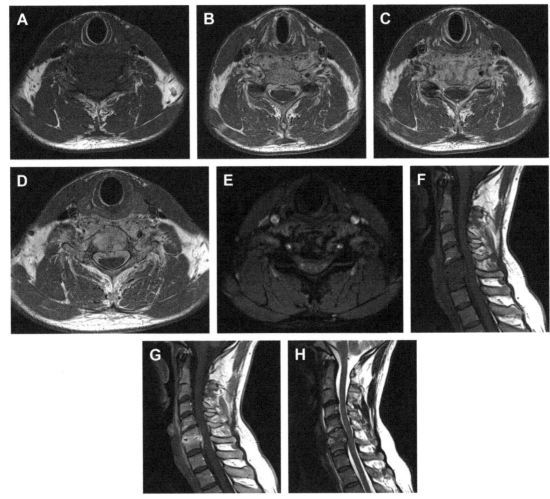

Fig. 3. Patient 3, a 43-year-old man with progressive pain in the neck for 2 months after a home renovation project. (A) MR imaging axial T1, (B–D) axial CE T1, (E) axial gradient-recalled echo (GRE) T2*, (F) sagittal T1, (G) sagittal CE T1, (H) sagittal T2. The patient had a cervical epidural infiltration twice. Congenital vertebral ankylosis C2-C3. Spondylodiscitis C6-C7 with irregular contours of the subchondral bone, loss of vertebral height, and contrast enhancement of the disk and the bone marrow of C6 and C7. There is extensive phlegmon formation in the anterior epidural space, around the foraminal nerve roots and in the prevertebral space. The patient was treated with conservative antibiotic therapy.

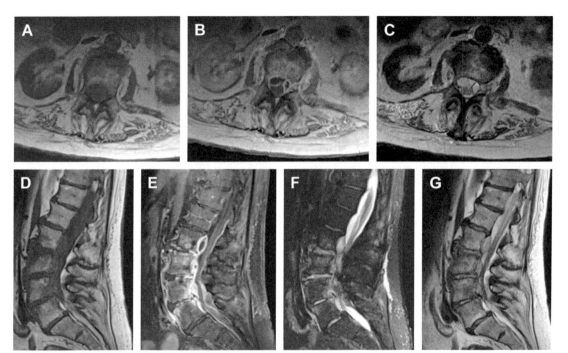

Fig. 4. Patient 4, a 65-year-old woman with progressive low back pain for 4 weeks. MR imaging (*A, B*) axial CE T1, (*C*) axial T2, (*D*) sagittal T1, (*E*) sagittal CE T1, (*F*) sagittal STIR, (*G*) sagittal T2. The MR imaging shows thick rim-enhancing collections in the anterior epidural space in four consecutive levels, suggestive for empyema. Also there is a multilevel spondylodiscitis from L2-L3 up to L4-L5. The patient was operated on, and *Mycobacterium tuberculosis* was confirmed on pathology.

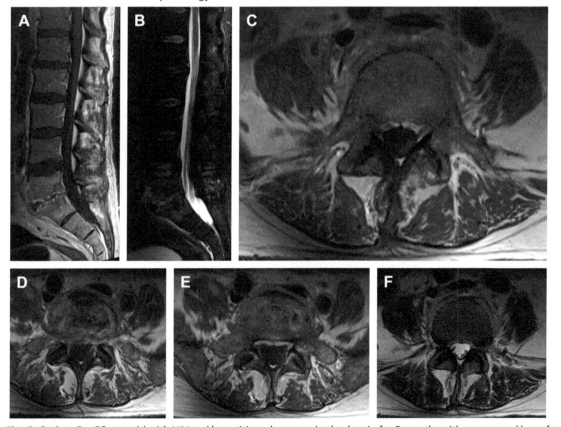

Fig. 5. Patient 5, a 56 year old with HIV and hepatitis and progressive back pain for 3 months with sensory and loss of strength. MR imaging (*A*) sagittal CE T1, (*B*) sagittal STIR, (*C–E*) axial CE T1, (*F*) axial T2. Spondylodiscitis L5-S1 with irregular vertebral contours, edema, and abscess formation in the disk space and also in the right psoas. Also extravertebral phlegmon formation paravertebral and in the anterior epidural space and around the foraminal nerve roots.

and *Enterobacter* sp. Therefore, they can result more often in osteomyelitis (**Fig. 6**).[1,2,4,5,7]

Nonpyogenic infectious spinal infections are mostly caused by *M tuberculosis* and do not produce proteolytic enzymes. Therefore, they progress more slowly, resulting in large abscess formation in the epidural and paravertebral tissues with multilevel involvement and soft tissue calcifications, intraosseous abscess formation, and initially sparing of the intervertebral disks. TB spondylodiscitis primarily is located at the thoracic level, probably because of mediastinal pathologic lymph nodes. Also these infections can cause extensive deformation of the spine by multilevel compression fractures (**Fig. 7**).[1,2,4,5,7]

Spinal epidural abscess formation is a serious complication. They are often not fatal as an entity; however, because of complications, mortality rates are 10% to 30%, depending on the literature. Also paraplegia or quadriplegia is frequent. The degree of neurologic loss is often greater than explained by mechanical compression alone, suggesting arterial occlusion, venous thrombosis, vasculitis, or by direct toxic effects. It affects 4% to 38% of the cases of nonpostoperative

spondylodiscitis. It usually occurs in the anterior epidural space and can give rise to the so-called curtain sign (see **Fig. 1**); however, this is a nonspecific finding and can also occur in tumoral lesions. Spondylodiscitis affecting the more cephalad regions of the spine is more prone to developing epidural abscesses, with an increasing risk of developing serious neurologic deficit (see **Figs. 4** and **7**).[1,2,4,5,7,10] Therapy mostly entails surgical decompression and/or long-term antibiotic treatment.

FRACTURES AND MALFORMATION

The vertebral body primarily serves as a load-bearing structure. Destruction of the disk and subchondral bone causes a decrease in disk height, whereas long-lasting infection can cause reactive sclerosis, new bone formation with osteophytes, and even bony ankylosis. Therefore, gradual destruction of the intervertebral disks, cortex, and trabeculae can cause local instability and collapse of the vertebral body (**Figs. 8–10**).

Over time these structural changes can gradually result in an increase in deformity with

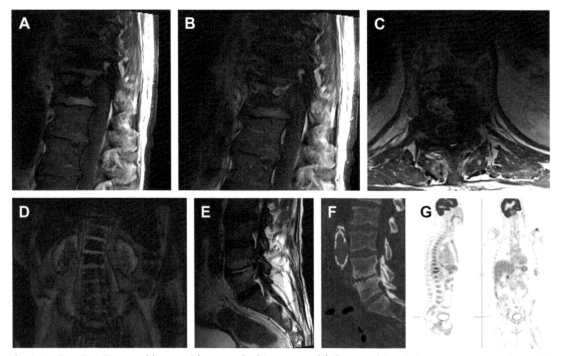

Fig. 6. Patient 6, a 62-year-old man with a vascular history, renal failure, and *Staphylococcus aureus* endocarditis with septicemia. MR imaging (*A, B*) sagittal CE T1, (*C*) axial CE T1, (*D*) coronal GRE scout, (*E*) sagittal T2, (*F*) computed tomography (CT) scan with sagittal reconstructions, and (*G*) fluorodeoxyglucose PET scan. Because of nonspecific back pain, an MR imaging was performed. Spondylodiscitis Th11-Th12 with extensive paravertebral and retroperitoneal phlegmon and abscess formation over three thoracic levels. Intraosseous abscesses in a vertebral body of Th12. Degeneration L5-S1 with deformation of the spine and a right-sided scoliosis, as seen on the coronal scout image. PET scan shows increased uptake at Th11-Th12, but not at L5-S1.

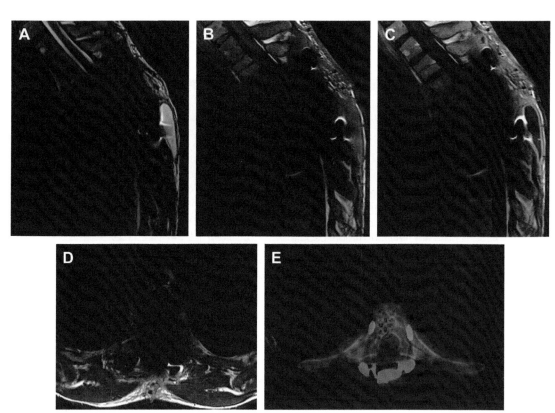

Fig. 7. Patient 7, a 45-year-old man with known Pott disease in the thoracic spine with paravertebral abscess formation, expanding over four levels. MR imaging (A) sagittal T2, (B) sagittal T1, (C) sagittal CE T1, (D) axial CE T1, and (E) single-photon emission CT scan (with technetium [99m] labeled white blood cells). Unstable destruction of two vertebrae, stabilization with posterior fusion, postoperative collection under the laminectomy defect. Bone scintigraphy shows no increased uptake of technetium [99m], proof of a so-called cold abscess, suggesting an infection with *Mycobacterium tuberculosis*.

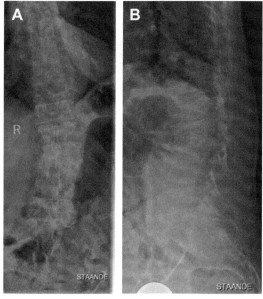

Fig. 8. Patient 8, a 74-year-old woman with a history of Pott disease (*Mycobacterium bovis*) 6 years earlier and now with complaints of chronic low back pain. Conventional radiography (A) anteroposterior and (B) lateral. Extensive destruction of three vertebrae with resulting kyphosis, ankylosis, and left-sided scoliosis.

malalignment, such as kyphosis and gibbus formation, scoliosis, and instability with neurologic deficit and even disability. The guidelines for the restoration of spinal instability are similar to those applied in direct trauma.[5]

Extensive spine deformation and malalignment is frequently encountered in the endemic areas of *M tuberculosis*, because of the multilevel involvement and slow progression over years (see Fig. 7).

NEUROLOGIC COMPLICATIONS

In the acute phase spondylodiscitis can lead to spinal and foraminal stenosis. Mechanical compression is the most common cause of functional compromise of the spinal cord. Ischemic compromise of the spinal cord is seldom seen. Phlegmon and abscess formation can cause nerve root irritation, leading to radicular pain, such as pain in the neck, chest, or abdomen (see Figs. 3 and 5).[1,10]

Only rarely does the infection spread to the meninges and then is called spinal meningitis.[1] It is caused by hematogenous spread and by the contiguous foci of infection. It is mostly diagnosed in the cerebrospinal fluid. Radiologically it is only

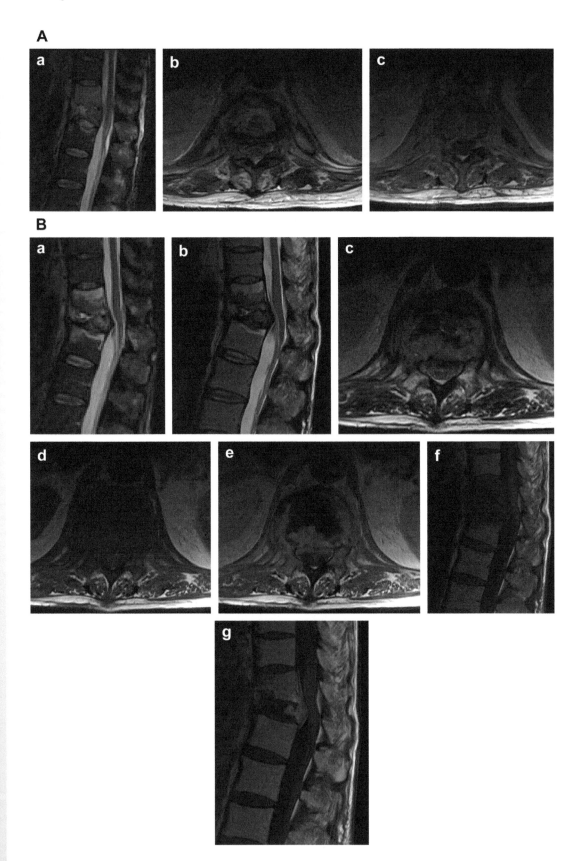

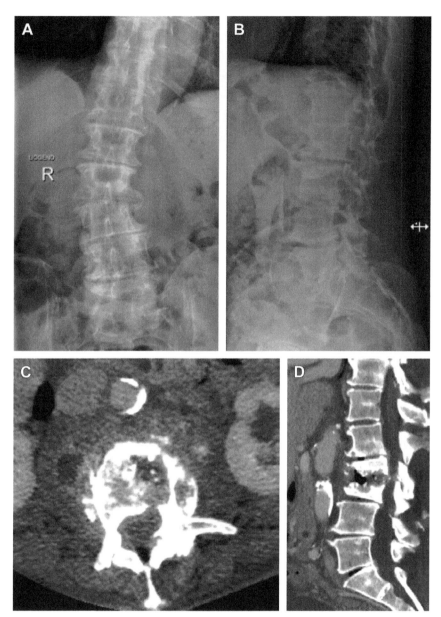

Fig. 10. Patient 10, a 78 year old presenting with disturbance of the gait, low back pain, and pain in the right leg. Conventional radiograph of the lumbar spine (A) anteroposterior and (B) lateral and CE CT scan (C) axial and (D) sagittal. The conventional radiograph shows deformation of the lumbar spine, extensive subchondral sclerosis anterior in L2-L3, and scoliosis. Because of infection without origin an MR imaging was performed and shows spondylodiscitis L2-L3 with a psoas abscess on the right side, phlegmon formation paravertebral with calcifications, and destruction of the adjacent vertebrae with lumbar kyphosis. *Candida albicans* was found.

Fig. 9. Patient 9, a 54-year-old man, known with intravenous drug abuse, with back pain for 2 months, who felt something when lifting a load. Hospitalized because of pneumonia. (A) First MR imaging at time 0 (a) sagittal STIR, (b) axial T2, (c) axial CE T1. (B) Second MR imaging 4 weeks later (a) sagittal STIR, (b) sagittal T2, (c) axial T2, (d) axial T1, (e) axial CE T1, (f) sagittal T1, (g) sagittal CE T1. Spondylitis with fracture of Th12 and also destruction of Th11. Progressive destruction and retropulsion of the posterior wall of the vertebra in the spinal canal with stenosis. Bilateral abscess formation in the psoas muscle.

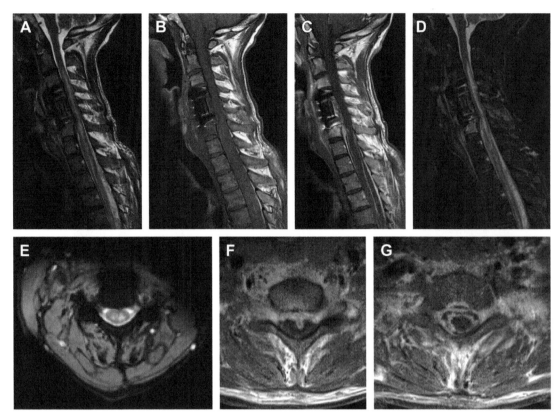

Fig. 11. Patient 11, a 45-year-old man. MR imaging (*A*) sagittal T2, (*B*) sagittal T1, (*C*) sagittal CE T1, (*D*) sagittal STIR, (*E*) axial GRE T2*, (*F, G*) axial CE T1. Corporectomy C5 for spinal stenosis with bilateral cervicobrachialgia. Sensory loss of the thoracic wall, urinary incontinence, and retention and paralytic ileus. Loss of strength in the left arm. MR imaging shows phlegmon in the anterior epidural space on C5-C6, in continuity with the dural sac. The axial CE CT shows an abnormal connection and defect in the dural sac with enhancement of the leptomengeal lining of the myelum. Thickening and T2 hyperintense signal of the myelum on the underlying levels, sign of myelopathy.

seen on postcontrast T1-weighted MR imaging, which shows enhancement of the meningeal surface (Fig. 11). However, the severity of contrast enhancement does not correlate with the course of the disease, as in the case of the more common intracranial counterpart.[1]

After the acute phase it can lead to arachnoiditis, a relative frequent sequel of lumbar spondylodiscitis. This is thickening and clumping of nerve roots in the cauda equina with adhesion at the peripheral dura. Patients have nonspecific complaints, such as chronic low back pain and leg pain, simulating spinal stenosis and polyneuropathy. Less commonly it gives rise to paraparesis, hypoesthesia, gait disorder, and bowel and bladder dysfunction (Fig. 12).

Spinal cord involvement or septic myelitis caused by spondylitis is very rare and is mainly transmitted by hematogenous spread of viral cardiopulmonary foci. Congenital abnormalities, such as diastematomyelia, are predisposing factors. It can cause weakness and progressive sensory disturbances in the extremities and even incontinence. However, because the diagnosis is often delayed because of the insidious course, it often leads to paralysis, up to 58% depending on the literature. It can even result in syringomyelia or even atrophy of the myelum (Fig. 13).[1] MR imaging shows a variable degree of edema, swelling, contrast enhancement, and even abscess formation in the myelum (see Fig. 11).

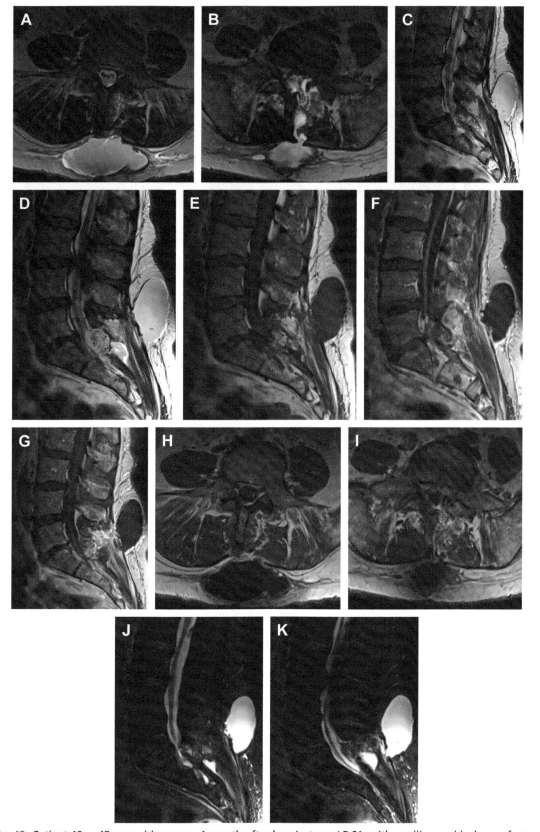

Fig. 12. Patient 12, a 45-year-old woman, 1 month after herniectomy L5-S1, with swelling and leakage of cerebrospinal fluid through the operation scar. MR imaging (*A, B*) axial T2, (*C, D*) sagittal T2, (*E*) sagittal T1, (*F, G*) sagittal CE T1, (*H, I*) axial CE T1, (*J, K*) sagittal STIR. MR imaging shows a large collection in the postoperative region, in continuity with the dura and abnormal thickening and enhancement of the radices in the cauda equina, suggestive of arachnoiditis and neuritis.

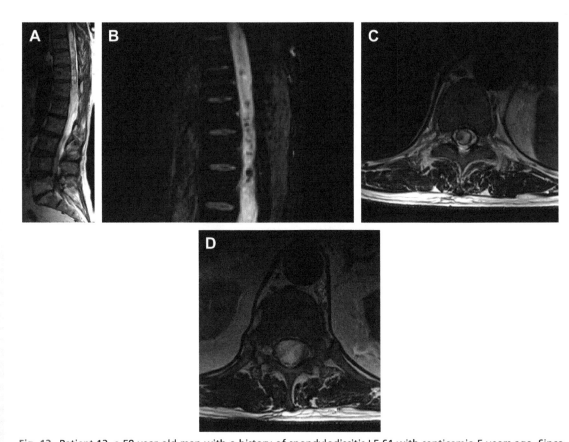

Fig. 13. Patient 13, a 58-year-old man with a history of spondylodiscitis L5-S1 with septicemia 5 years ago. Since then progressive sensory loss in the legs expanding to the thorax and now also urinary retention. MR imaging (*A*) sagittal T2, (*B*) sagittal GRE T2*, (*C, D*) axial T2. The MR imaging shows extensive myelitis distal in the myelum with susceptibility artifacts on the gradient echo, probably because of blood degradation products. More distally is seen thickening and peripheral position of the cauda nerve roots because of arachnoiditis.

SUMMARY

Spinal infection is spectrum of diseases involving the bone, disks, and/or ligaments. There has been written evidence of the complications since ancient Egyptian civilization, with mostly spinal deformation. Treatment was mainly based on managing the deformity.

Mortality rates were around 70% before the use of antibiotics.[5] However, because of the indolent course, there is still an important delay in diagnosis with a mortality rate between 2% and 11%, according to the literature.

A fast diagnosis remains crucial and the cornerstone remains MR imaging and a high clinical suspicion. Until recent years, complications of spinal infections were mostly caused by *M tuberculosis*, with extensive multilevel deformation of the spine. With the rise of all kinds of spinal interventions, more and more spinal infections are iatrogenic, up to 20% to 30%.

In all infections, there is a balance between the virulence of an infection and the immunity of a host. In the last decade there has been a significant rise in the immunocompromised patient population, making spinal infection a growing and changing group of conditions, and diagnosis based on imaging more challenging.

The most common complication is the direct extraspinal spread of infection, mostly to the epidural space. Neurologic complications overall are not often encountered and mostly caused by radicular irritation. Long-term spinal disability is around 33%, with only 3% with severe disability.[11]

REFERENCES

1. Lury K, Smith JK, Castillo M. Imaging of spinal infections. Semin Roentgenol 2006;41:363–79.
2. Tali ET. Spinal infections. Eur J Radiol 2014;50: 120–33.

3. Mylona E, Samarkos M, Kakalou E, et al. Pyogenic vertebral osteomyelitis: a systematic review of clinical characteristics. Semin Arthritis Rheum 2008;39:10–7.

4. Cottle L, Riordan T. Infectious spondylodiscitis. J Infect 2008;56:401–12.

5. Lehovsky J. Pyogenic vertebral osteomyelitis/disc infection. Baillieres Best Pract Res Clin Rheumatol 1999;13(1):59–75.

6. Modic MT, Feiglin DH, Piraino DW, et al. Vertebral osteomyelitis: assessment using MR. Radiology 1985;185(157):157–66.

7. Dagirmanjijan A, Schils J, McHenry M, et al. MR imaging of vertebral osteomyelitis revisited. AJR Am J Roentgenol 1996;167:1539–43.

8. Ledermann HP, Schweitzer ME, Morrisson WB, et al. MR imaging findings in spinal infections: rules or myths? Radiology 2003;228:506–14.

9. Friedman JA, Maher CO, Quast LM, et al. Spontaneous disc space infections. Surg Neurol 2002;57: 81–6.

10. Tang HJ, Lin HJ, Liu YC, et al. Spinal epidural abscess: experience with 46 patients and evaluation of prognostic factors. J Infect 2002;45: 76–81.

11. Solis Garcia del Pozo J, Vives Soto M, Solera J. Vertebral osteomyelitis: long-term disability assessment and prognostic factors. J Infect 2007; 54:129–34.

Index

Note: Page numbers of article titles are in **boldface** type.

neuroimaging.theclinics.com

Neuroimag Clin N Am 25 (2015) 323–325
http://dx.doi.org/10.1016/S1052-5149(15)00023-4
1052-5149/15/$ – see front matter © 2015 Elsevier Inc. All rights reserved.

Printed and bound by CPI Group (UK) Ltd, Croydon, CR0 4YY

03/10/2024

01040382-0015